THE M&S
HOME
EMERGENCY
HANDBOOK
&
FIRST-AID
GUIDE

THE M&S
HOME
EMERGENCY
HANDBOOK
&
FIRST-AID
GUIDE

FRED KERNER

CANADIAN CATALOGUING IN PUBLICATION DATA

Kerner, Fred, 1921-
    Home emergency handbook and first-aid guide

ISBN 0-7710-4478-X

1. Home accidents.   2. Home accidents —
Prevention. 3. Dwellings — Security measures.
4. First aid in illness and injury.   I. Title.

TX 150.K47 1990   363.13   C90-093058-6

DESIGN: ArtPlus Limited / Brant Cowie
PAGE MAKE UP: ArtPlus Limited / Valerie Van Volkenburg
ILLUSTRATIONS: Paul McCusker

MCCLELLAND & STEWART INC.
The Canadian Publishers
481 University Avenue
Toronto, Ontario
M5G 2E9

Printed and bound in Canada

Contents

CHAPTER 1

Fire: The Ever-Present Danger

YOU WANT TO HAVE the proverbial safe-and-sound feeling in your own home. Yet, within that "safety zone" there is an omnipresent threat: fire.

Few things trigger as much fear in people as the shouted word, "Fire!" That cry, in a public place, can cause a level of panic that must be experienced to be believed. In a matter of moments, fire can destroy your years of efforts to provide a safe, comfortable shelter for your family. In a matter of moments, fire can literally tear down, rip apart, and raze to the ground structural monuments that were built to survive for centuries.

Of all of nature's destructive forces none seems so pervasive as the force of fire. A wall of water propelled by hurricane-force winds is itself awesome. When city streets crack and buildings tumble at the height of an earthquake even seeing is almost not believing. The bone-chilling experience of a building exploding around you as a tornado passes by is something you would rather watch on television, far from the danger zone. But all these natural tragedies can be – indeed, often are – followed by *fire*. When a catastrophe strikes, all materials that can burn are subject to being set aflame in any of a dozen different ways: torn electric lines sparking, broken gas lines igniting, shredded fuel tanks and their escaping fumes exploding. Substances you never thought would burn suddenly disintegrate in a wall of red and orange heat that chokes off the oxygen you need to breathe; that scorches the largest organ of your body, the skin; that turns to ashes your every possession.

In the haven of your own home, fire is an ever-present threat. But there are ways to minimize the fire hazards in your house.

Combustion and Explosive Mixtures

We all think we know what "combustion," "flammable," and "inflammable" mean: they mean burning or burnable. But to understand how to protect yourself you should also learn what happens in combustion, in other words, *why* things burn.

When we speak of combustion, we are speaking about a chemical reaction: oxidation. Burning is the *rapid* combination of certain materials with oxygen at high temperatures. It may be shocking to you to understand that oxygen, the very gas we breathe to sustain life, is the same chemical that sustains fire.

Wood, paper, and cloth, for example, will combine with oxygen from the atmosphere if the temperature of the material rises to a certain point. The burning substance will usually turn black because the residue left after burning is mostly carbon, and carbon is black.

The flames you see rising from the burning material are actually burning gases. Carbon dioxide, carbon monoxide, and steam are the major by-products of combustion. These gases, rather than fire, often cause death or injury because their production decreases the supply of oxygen necessary for life. Some super-heated gases are not even visible, but they are killers nevertheless. In a large fire they precede the visible gases and, if inhaled, sear the lungs.

Most of the materials we think of as dangerously flammable – such as gasoline, alcohol, and the like – are made from various combinations of carbon, hydrogen, and oxygen. These materials include hydrocarbons and carbohydrates. In order for there to be combustion of these materials, three things must be present: oxygen, fuel, and sufficient heat to maintain the fire.

Heat need not come from a spark or flame. Spontaneous combustion – a fire starting without any external cause – can occur, for example, when oily rags or greasy clothing build up heat from a chemical reaction. Storing such rags in a sealed metal container that restricts the available oxygen can prevent this type of fire.

Different substances require different levels of temperature for burning to begin. Paper and cloth usually burn easily. There are two reasons for this:

- The temperature at which they combine with oxygen is relatively low when compared to the temperatures at which other materials combine with oxygen.
- They are constructed in a thin layer so that small amounts of the material well supplied by oxygen are available to a heat source; holding a flame to them for just a few seconds is sufficient to increase the temperature of a small portion to the burning point.

Certain hydrocarbons (e.g., gasoline, naphtha, kerosene) contain only carbon and hydrogen. These two substances are even easier to ignite. What's worse, they burn so rapidly that they actually "flash" into flame. The temperature at which this occurs is called the "flash point."

Because the vapours of gasoline, naphtha, and some other fuels and solvents are heavier than air, they will drift along the floor of a room until they reach a source of ignition. Then they flash back to the main body of the liquid and/or vapour and ignite it explosively.

Explosive Mixtures

An explosion takes place when there is extremely rapid combustion, especially if this happens in a confined space. So any substance that is flammable can also be explosive when it is mixed with air or oxygen in the proper proportions. The "ideal" conditions for an explosion occur when any highly flammable substance is mixed with a sufficient amount of air so that the entire substance can burst into flame at the same instant. Under these conditions, the gases generated in the combustion process develop in large quantity, at great speed, and with violent results.

Some substances, such as gasoline and paint thinners, can satisfy these conditions very easily. Even at normal room temperatures they are constantly evaporating and – given enough time – can fill a room with their vapours. Striking a match, or even creating a spark near such a substance, can cause an explosion or fire. Such ignition *cannot* occur in a *closed* can that contains a flammable liquid, due to the lack of oxygen.

CAUTION

Not only flammable liquids can explode in this way. Dust, large quantities of flour, or sawdust, when mixed with air, also can explode. In these instances the heat caused by friction – the tiny particles rubbing against each other – can ignite the material. Any other solid flammable material that hangs suspended in the air like a gas can similarly explode.

Electricity – The Invisible Power Source

Everyone has heard about Benjamin Franklin and his experiments flying a kite that had a brass key attached to the cord. That was one of the earliest experiments with electricity; and old Ben was playing with fire. He could easily have sustained a fatal shock, though he had no idea of the danger when he made his famous experiment.

Today, we understand the danger of electrical shock; we discuss that household hazard fully in the next chapter. But we often fail to realize that electricity can be a sudden source of *fire*, too. Strangely enough, there is little excuse for anyone to be exposed to the hazard of electrical fire because we have ample knowledge about the dangers of electricity. If a fire should start due to faulty wiring or any other electrical cause, never, *never*, **never** use water to try to extinguish the flames. There is a serious shock hazard in pouring water on a fire.

Home with the Range

Someone in your home probably prepares three meals a day, and by that token it is safe to say that your cooking range and/or microwave oven is one of your most important appliances. They also are the most hazardous appliances in your home.

You should be aware that . . .
- Vapours from contact cement, gasoline, cleaning fluids, or other flammable liquids can be ignited by the pilot light on your kitchen gas range.
- An electric burner coil can reach a temperature of more than 1,000°F (537.7°C) and that's a level of heat that can ignite your clothing even after the coil has been turned off.
- Flammable fabrics, such as towels, dish rags, or curtains, can be ignited merely by being used or hung *near* a gas or electric range.
- Most kitchen range fires happen when clothing, particularly a loose-fitting sleeve, catches fire while the victim is cooking or reaching across a range.
- An oven door can get hot enough to burn a youngster who might fall or lean against it. It can be particularly dangerous for a child just learning to walk who may use the door for support. The child is often unable to let go before suffering a burn.

So while the range or oven can be a danger to you – it can be an especially serious hazard to children. Keep small children out of the kitchen when the oven is in use; and keep a close eye on them when you are cooking on the stove-top. Fires also occur when the range is not in use for cooking: for example, when a child climbs onto the range; when someone leans over the range to reach a shelf or cabinet; when someone leans against the range for warmth; when the controls are accidently turned on; and when hot oven doors are touched.

If you are buying a new range, here are some important things to consider before you make your choice:

- Are the controls on the range out of the reach of young children?
- Do the knobs turn through a progression of temperature settings before coming to maximum heat?
- Are the controls placed so that you don't have to reach across the burners to turn the range on and off?
- If the range is electric, does it have signal lamps that warn when the burners are on?
- Does the range comply with the current voluntary standards for electric and gas ranges?

With regard to the last question, have the dealer show you the information that indicates the range you selected meets electrical, gas, and/or thermal standards.

YOUR MICROWAVE OVEN: IS ITS RADIATION DANGEROUS?

When microwave ovens first became available for use at home, some models leaked radiation in amounts that caused alarm. In the last decade or so, however, the design of these ovens has greatly improved and the risk of excessive leakage is low.

It is important to know that microwave radiation is not the same as nuclear radiation. Nuclear radiation is a far more intense form of electromagnetic energy and is discussed in Chapters Seven and Eight. Suffice it to note that the x-rays and gamma rays from nuclear radiation can harm living cells even at relatively low levels. But the heating effect of microwaves can damage human tissue as well as cook food.

Medical experts suggest that the lens of the eye, the testicles, and the developing fetus would be most vulnerable to excessive microwave radiation. But as far as microwave ovens are concerned, there seems to be no evidence of hazard.

How much leakage is there in newer models? Tests have shown that less than half the amount permitted by safety standards bodies has been found in the worst cases. But it should be noted that the radiation a person may be exposed to while working around the kitchen will depend on distance from the oven and the time spent around it, as well as on how much leakage there may be.

Radiation intensity declines sharply the fartl.er away a person is from the oven. And since you are unlikely to just stand in one spot, but move around the room and even leave it from time to time, exposure at most may last for a minute or two.

To be absolutely on the safe side, follow these rules:
• Keep a reasonable distance from the oven when it's on.
• Don't make a habit of peering into the window for long periods.
• Make sure food residue does not build up around the door seal so that it doesn't close tightly.
• Never use a swing-down door as a shelf.

REMEMBER: If the door, its seal, or its hinges become damaged, do not use the oven until it's repaired.

When you buy your range, why not buy a fire extinguisher as well, one that has been approved by a qualified testing service.

CAUTION

Read the instructions that come with an extinguisher *before* you have a fire and keep it handy, but not within the potential fire area.

Stove-Top Fires

To prevent stove-top fires, keep the area around your kitchen range free of grease. And don't heat grease until it smokes, because you'll increase the chance of it splattering and catching fire.

If you should have a fire:
Do turn the burner off.
Do cover the pan with a lid carefully. Slide it on from the front, deflecting the flames away from you.
Don't carry the pan to the sink.
Don't ever put water on a grease fire.

If you can't cover the pan, use a dry chemical or carbon dioxide fire extinguisher. If you don't have an extinguisher, baking soda can be used. You must have enough of it handy to smother the fire entirely. Use the container as a shaker, starting at the front and working back, as the soda covers the flames. Try to spread the powder gently so as not to scatter the flaming grease.

Flammable Liquids

Flammable liquids are liquids that will burn. Furthermore, most flammable liquids will evaporate much more readily than water. It is this ability to change from a liquid to a gaseous (vapour) state that makes flammable liquids so dangerous when they mix with air. The majority of these liquids are distilled from crude oil. They include gasoline, kerosene, "mineral spirits," benzine (also called dry-cleaning fluid), and others.

Their "volatility" (the temperature at which they can vapourize and explode) is reckoned by their "flash points." Gasoline, for example, emits flammable vapours even at air temperatures below the freezing point of water (32°F or 0°C).

As we indicated, flammable liquids are not only a fire hazard, they are also dangerously explosive. Here are some important points to remember about flammable liquids:

- Vapours from flammable liquids are heavier than air. Therefore, they can flow invisibly along the ground and can be ignited by a far-off flame, spark, or heat source. The vapour trail can act as a wick!
- Flammable liquids should be used *only* in well-ventilated areas.
- Even in cold weather, vapours can escape from an open flammable-liquid container.
- Gasoline-powered equipment must be turned off and *cooled* before being refueled, to prevent ignition of gasoline vapour.
- Never try to extinguish a flammable-liquid fire with water: it can cause the fire to spread or to explode.
- Local regulations often prohibit the storage of large amounts of gasoline in inhabited buildings.
- Never use or keep a flammable liquid near a source of flame or heat.
- Don't add liquid fuel to a charcoal fire after it has started, because flames could travel up to the container and cause it to explode. Never use gasoline to start a charcoal fire.
- Never store gasoline in your home or car. Flammable liquids must be kept in a well-ventilated area.
- If you must siphon gasoline, use a hand-operated pump; don't start the siphoning action with your mouth.
- Gasoline should be stored in tightly capped, appropriately labelled safety cans that have flame arresters and pressure-relief valves – never in glass or plastic jugs.
- Keep flammable liquids out of the reach of children.
- Use only Class "B" fire extinguishers (foam, carbon dioxide, or dry chemical) to put out flammable-liquid fires.
- Never incinerate, heat, or puncture pressurized containers.
- Read the directions before using a spot remover, and avoid using it near a heat source.
- Never use gasoline as a cleaning agent.

CAUTION

Oil-soaked rags or clothing are especially flammable.
Always store them in a covered metal container.

If you should spill a flammable liquid, clean up the spill immediately. Better yet, use a safety can; it won't spill when tipped.

Be *very* careful with charcoal fires. Light them only outdoors and treat the starter fluid as cautiously as you would gasoline.

Whenever possible, you should choose products that are non-flammable and non-toxic. Read labels carefully and follow the directions for use and storage. This warning takes into consideration that some flammable liquids have a legitimate reason to be in the home. However, most do not.

Why not do a house check immediately to determine which of the following liquids you have around your home? If you have any of them, are you using them and storing them properly?

GASOLINE. If you must store gasoline (for a power lawn mower, etc.), keep no more than a gallon or two in a cool location (such as your garage), but only in a suitably marked, tightly closed container.

BENZINE. If you keep benzine in the house as a dry-cleaning fluid or as a fluid for your cigarette lighter, you should keep the smallest quantity possible on hand. Use a tightly stoppered container to store it away securely in a cool place. *Beware* of benzene (spelled with an "e," not an "i"), otherwise known as benzol. Benzene is a solvent used in the chemical industry and is a very serious fire and health hazard. Do not use or store it under any circumstances.

DENATURED ALCOHOL (also called rubbing alcohol). This may be required for some uses in the home. While it is not quite as dangerous as some of the hydrocarbons, it is nonetheless highly flammable and should be used and stored with as much caution as any other flammable liquid.

PAINT SPRAYS, PAINT REMOVERS, SYNTHETIC THINNERS, QUICK-DRYING PAINTS. These can be extremely dangerous products because they evaporate easily, and their vapours will accumulate in a closed room. Use them out-of-doors only, and store them in labelled, tightly capped metal containers. Do not breathe the vapours.

Space Heaters

Even with central heating we still need to warm individual rooms from time to time. And to do this, we use either space heaters or fireplaces. Today's small room-heaters use either gas, oil, or electricity. And solid fuel is burned in fireplaces of various kinds.

The gas-fired room heater gives off a pleasant red glow, can be vented or unvented, and works on the principle of a porcelain device that stores and radiates heat provided by gas flames. Its potential hazards are fire, poisonous fumes, explosion, clothing ignition, and hot surfaces.

The oil-heated space heater usually burns kerosene. It may be unvented or vented through a stove pipe or chimney. This open-flame type of heater is popular in rural areas. Its potential hazards are fire, clothing ignition, flash fire, poisonous fumes, explosion, and hot surfaces.

The electric room heater has long, narrow coils that generate warmth. They can be automatic (thermostatic), and they often have a fan, which disseminates the heat, and may or may not have separate manual controls. The potential hazards of electric heaters are shock, fire, clothing ignition, and hot surfaces.

If you use any of the three types mentioned above, here are some pointers:
• If your heater is unvented, keep a window or door at least partially open.

- If you have a gas heater, light the match *before* you turn on the gas.
- Teach your children about the dangers of playing near a space heater.
- Make sure your space heater is inspected, cleaned, and adjusted regularly.
- Never use an electric space heater near a water source, such as in the bathroom or in the kitchen.
- Make sure there is at least three feet of space between your heater and any flammables in the room (draperies, furniture, bedding, magazine rack, etc.).
- Keep your space heater out of the "heavy traffic" areas of the room.
- Keep the damper open while fuel is burning.
- Make sure all ashes are cooled before you dispose of them.
- *Never* fall asleep with an unvented heater operating.
- *Never* store flammable liquids near your heater.
- If your heater has an open flame, make sure there is a metal screen around it.

Fireplaces

A fireplace consists of three main parts: the *fireplace* itself, in which fuel is actually burned; the *chimney*, through which smoke and hot gases escape; and the *hearth*, a kind of apron in front of the fireplace, made of brick and some other non-flammable material.

You may think of a chimney as a structure that extends above the roof of the house. It actually includes the part below the roof, too. Inside the chimney, there is a passageway called a *flue* through which smoke and hot gases travel. Since these gases are at or above the temperature of the logs burning in the fireplace, the chimney must be lined with a fire-resistant material. In modern chimneys, a material called "firebrick" is generally used for this purpose; or a fire-resistant liner is incorporated into the flue. For added protection, firebrick is frequently used to line the interior walls of the fireplace as well.

Smoke and heated gases rise by convection in the chimney. This draws air from the room into the fireplace and through the logs, creating a draft. The effect grows steadily. The greater the fire, the more gases are produced, the more fresh air is drawn in, the hotter the fire grows until the fire literally begins to roar.

As you can see, such a process could cause a fire to get out of hand. To prevent this from happening, the chimney has a "damper" just above the fireplace. This is a metal plate controlled by a handle that closes off some or all of the flue in the chimney. Thus the draft is reduced and the combustion in the fireplace is controlled.

As the principal control of the fireplace, the damper must be used properly. If it is kept entirely shut the fire will become oxygen-starved and it is likely to send smoke and gases into the room instead of up the chimney. The damper must be set so that while the fire draws smoke and gases up the chimney, at the same time it draws air into the fireplace from the room.

And the fire must not be allowed to get so hot and roaring that it begins to throw sparks across the room. That is why a *screen* made of wire or special glass should be kept in front of the fireplace. A blazing fire can be beautiful. But if it's not carefully understood and monitored, it can also be a killer.

Here are some valuable pointers to remember if you like using your fireplace:
- Sparks leaping from an open fireplace can ignite anything flammable in a room.
- Artificial logs, made of compressed sawdust and wax, should be handled differently (used one at a time, and *not* stacked) from natural logs because they generate more heat.
- Never mix artificial and natural logs in the same fire.
- Charcoal and plastic packing materials (like polystyrene) burned in a poorly ventilated fireplace generate poisons and deadly gases (such as carbon monoxide).
- Using gasoline and other highly volatile, flammable solvents to encourage a fire in a fireplace causes the emission of

invisible vapours that are themselves flammable – and they are explosive!

REMEMBER: relatively safe kerosene or fuel oil will behave like gasoline when vapourized by the heat of the fire.

And if, in spite of all your precautions, the unexpected occurs and a spark ignites something flammable in a room, have a fire extinguisher close at hand. A pressurized water-charged extinguisher is best for this type of fire. (See chart on page 24.)

Flammable Fabrics

Fabric and flame don't mix. And if you keep that simple dictum in mind, you can reduce the incidence of fire in the home. The clothing you wear, the upholstery on your furniture, the draperies and curtains on your windows, the linens on your bed, the towels you use in the kitchen and bathroom – these are all flammable materials that ignite easily when they are exposed to flame.

When you can, use flame-resistant fabrics. Each fabric and garment is labelled with its own special care instructions, because different laundering methods may change the flame-retardant characteristics. So be sure to look for, and follow, all special care instructions when laundering flame-resistant fabrics.

Research has shown us that:
• Children set their clothing on fire most often while playing with matches or lighters.
• If you spill lighter fluid on your clothing and then light a match or a cigarette lighter, the flame is likely to ignite the vapours of the spilled fluid.
• A woman's clothing is most often ignited when she is cooking.
• A man's clothing is most often ignited when he is burning trash, using flammable liquids to clean, or working with machinery.
• If draperies, beds, upholstered furniture, or other household items catch fire, the heavy smoke and gases that are generated can cause death.

Safety with Matches

It is important to remember that matches that have been extinguished, but not cooled, can cause fires if they come into contact with something flammable. It is equally important to be aware that the ignition compounds on matchsticks are sometimes applied unevenly, so that when lit the matches can break apart and spit sparks and flame dangerously.

There are six different types of matches:

SAFETY MATCH. This type has the ingredients required for ignition divided between the match head and the striking surface. Therefore, it can only be lit if struck against the surface supplied for that purpose.

STRIKE-ANYWHERE or FRICTION MATCH. All the ignition ingredients are in the match head. As its name implies, it can be ignited by striking on any surface where friction is created.

WOODEN SAFETY or STRIKE-ON-BOX MATCH. An ignition head attached to a wooden splint. The splint is dipped in paraffin wax, which transfers the flame from the head to the splint.

DOUBLE-DIP or BIRD'S-EYE MATCH. A wooden strike-anywhere match, the head of which is "tipped" with an extremely sensitive striking material. These are safer than strike-anywhere matches.

BOOK MATCH. A safety match usually made from cardboard splints. The splints are joined at the base and stapled to a stiff paper cover.

FIREPLACE MATCH. Either "safety" or "strike-anywhere," the splints are longer so that they are convenient for awkward or dangerous situations like lighting a fireplace.

The following DOS and DON'TS of safety with matches are important if you wish to avoid fire accidents:

Do buy match books that have a striking surface on the back cover.

Do close the cover of the book or box *before* you strike a match.

Do make the motion of striking a match away from the body.

Do blow the match out as soon as you are finished using it.

Do check the match to make sure it isn't smouldering before you throw it away.

Do keep only one match book in the same pocket at any one time.

Do remind elderly family members and friends to use matches with caution.

Do store matches out of the reach of young children.

Do avoid "strike-anywhere" matches that will light when struck against any surface.

Do teach older children about the dangers of mishandling matches.

Don't let young children experiment with matches.

Don't hold the match any closer than an arm's length when you're striking it.

Don't buy or pick up match books with colourful covers that will attract children.

Don't use matches when something else – like driving a car – is distracting you.

Don't use matches around flammable liquids, especially gasoline.

Don't use a waste basket to discard a used match.

Don't light candles or cigarettes if you might fall asleep, leaving them burning.

Don't throw a match away until it is extinguished and cool to the touch.

While the convenience of a lighter is obvious, the dangers are less than apparent, perhaps because we have become so used to the gadgetry and because throw-away models are so inexpensive. There are a number of warnings you should be heedful of in this regard:

- When igniting a lighter, hold it away from you.
- Don't try to ignite your lighter when you are coughing.
- Don't use a lighter if you are driving a car; use the car's battery-fired lighter.
- Never put a lighter away until it has been extinguished.
- Don't use a lighter near flammable liquids.
- Check your lighter regularly for leakages.
- Fill a lighter out-of-doors or in a well-ventilated room to prevent fumes from building up.
- Clean up any spills, after filling your lighter, before you use it.
- Teach your children the dangers of using a lighter, just as you do about matches.

Nature's Own Fire Extinguisher

We are all accustomed to thinking of water as the natural fire extinguisher, and water is effective for a great many fires, but not for all. Fire extinction is accomplished by either or both of two ways: by cooling the burning substance to a point below its combustion temperature; and by denying the burning substance any oxygen. Water does both for many fires, but *not* for all.

A gasoline fire, for example, should not be touched by water. Gasoline is lighter than water and will float on top of it and continue to burn, while being spread farther by the water. Electrical fires should not be touched by water because water conducts electricity and can carry the electric current from broken wires to anyone who comes in contact with the water.

Still, both gasoline and electrical fires can be extinguished safely. So can most others. All you have to know is which type of fire extinguisher to use, and how to use it. The chart on the following page describes the different types of fire extinguishers commonly available, the kind of fires they are designed to extinguish, and the proper way to use them. Practise with your fire extinguisher in a safe location and be sure to have it recharged, even if it has only been partially used.

Fire Extinguishers for the Home

Suitable for use on:	Water		Dry Chemical			Carbon Dioxide	Halogenated Hydrocarbons	
	Pressurized Water	Pump Tank	Ordinary Sodium Bi-carbonate	Multi-Purpose	Potassium Bicarb. ("Purple K")		"Halon" 1301	"Halon" 1211
CLASS A FIRES: paper, wood, cloth, rubber, plastics, etc.	Yes	Yes	*	Yes	*	*	*	*
CLASS B FIRES: oil, gasoline, solvents, paint, cooking oil, grease, etc.	No	No	Yes	Yes	Yes	Yes	Yes	Yes
CLASS C FIRES: energized electrical wiring, equipment, and appliances	No	No	Yes	Yes	Yes	Yes	Yes	Yes
Usual size or capacity designation for extinguishers in the home	11⅓ litres (2½ gal.)	**	1 kilogram to 4.5 kilograms (2½ to 10 pounds)			4.5-6.75 kg (10-15 lbs.)	1-1.3 kilograms (2-3 lbs.)	

* Can be used to contain a fire, but may not extinguish it.

** No longer manufactured or commonly stocked.

Smoke Can Hurt

Many deaths and injuries due to home fires are caused by smoke – not by fire directly. And the statistics show another interesting fact: many of the deaths and injuries occur in fires that happen *at night*, while the victims are asleep. Obviously, a reliable way to awaken these sleepers before the smoke becomes unbreathably dense would help more people escape uninjured. And, of course, there is a way: the home smoke detector. Smoke detectors sense fire only a few minutes after it ignites, and they warn you several minutes before smoke becomes deadly. They provide an early warning that could enable you and your family to escape, and reduce the loss of your property.

There are two types to choose from:
• Ionization chamber detectors, which sense flaming fires quicker than photoelectric detectors.
• Photoelectric detectors, which sense smouldering fires quicker than ionization chamber detectors.

Which you should install actually depends on the size and layout of your home. You should call your local fire department to find out whether they will send someone around to suggest the best place to install detectors, and which type to install.

Since the primary job of a smoke detector is to awaken sleeping persons and warn them of urgent danger, the most critical location for the detector is as close as possible to the bedrooms in which your family sleeps. If two sleeping areas are separated by any significant distance, each should have its own detector.

Remember, there is more to surviving a home fire than waking up before it's too late. Just-awakened people, especially children, are often confused, and may panic. The safety of all may depend on knowing ahead of time what to do. Therefore, plan and practise for a safe escape.

Fire Drills

Home fire drills may sound silly, and a serious fire is no fun to talk about, but a little time spent selecting escape routes and practising what to do if the detector is triggered may save lives if fire ever occurs in your home.

- Walk through the main escape route several times. Try it in the dark or with your eyes closed. Memorize the number of steps between obstacles and turns. If a piece of furniture keeps getting in the way, change its position to clear the path.
- Plan alternate ways of escape from each room. If the main route would be blocked by fire or impenetrable smoke, how would each family member get out? If bedroom windows are too high to jump from safely, buy rope or chain escape-ladders to keep at a window in each bedroom.
- If you must go through a smoke-filled area, crawl on your hands and knees, with your head low to avoid breathing smoke.
- Before opening an inside door, touch the knob and the top of the door. If either feels hot, do not open the door. Fire on the other side might flash into your room.
- Agree on a place to meet outside the home, so you can count noses and be sure everyone is safe.
- Don't call the fire department from the burning home. Get out safely, then telephone from a neighbour's home or use an alarm box.
- Do not go back into the house or apartment until the fire-fighters have assured you that the fire is fully extinguished and the structure is sound.

2

Electricity: Living Safely With It

YOU FLICK A SWITCH to light a room. You turn a dial for instant entertainment. But what goes on behind that switch, that dial? What should you know to make your use of electricity as safe as possible? And how can you cope safely if there is a failure in your power source?

Before we explore the dangers of electricity in the home, it would be useful to understand the common terms of the science.

Electricity is a form of energy that can be used to do work. It is carried into our homes through protected (insulated) wires.

Voltage is the force that causes or directs current to flow, somewhat like the force of water pressure in a pipe. It is measured in volts.

Current is the rate of flow of an electrical charge, somewhat like the current of water in a stream. It is measured in amperes (amps). Fuses are constructed to burn out (melt, or "blow") if the current exceeds the amperage recommended for a particular electrical circuit (e.g., 15 amps, 30 amps, etc.).

Resistance is an "opposition" to electrical current, somewhat like the friction of a pipe to a flow of water in it.

Circuit is a continuous path of conductors through which a current can flow. A circuit may be a network of paths, such as the wiring in your house.

Circuit breaker is a device for opening and closing a circuit manually, and for opening a circuit automatically when there is an overload of current.

Charge is a basic electrical quantity that makes up an electrical current.

Ampere is the unit of measure of electric current.

Conductor is a substance through which current can flow when voltage is present. Examples of conductors: water, copper wire, the human body.

Insulator is a substance that is a poor conductor of electricity. Examples of insulators: glass, porcelain, rubber, plastics, ceramics, dry wood, and air. These things protect you from shock.

While the strength of the electricity used in your home for appliances is weak compared to the strength carried by power lines between the generators and their final destination, it is powerful enough to kill. Unless you know exactly what you are doing, *always proceed with caution.*

Don't be fooled when you compare voltage numbers. The voltage used in your home is 120 or 240. The 100,000 to 500,000 volts carried along high-voltage lines (you see them in urban and rural areas – those steel towers with huge arms that have wires running between them) seem vastly more dangerous.

Be warned: the amperage in the wires on the high-voltage lines is the same as in the wires leading to lights and appliances in your home. The different voltages refer to the amount of force needed to propel the electricity along the wires. So while only 120 to 140 volts of "push" are required to move electricity around in your home, the electricity surging through the wires to your hair dryer or food processor is as powerful as the electricity being carried along the "monster" poles outdoors.

Electricity leaves a generating station at about 20,000 volts. Then, to be distributed in your community, the voltage is decreased. Finally, small transformers right in your community (on the street, in fact) further reduce the voltage to carry the electricity into your home in the right proportion. From the street – either by means of underground lines or along utility-company poles – the electricity is carried to the *main switch box* in your home. This switch box is clearly marked with "on" and "off" positions. It controls all the power in the house.

Under normal daily use, the main switch is in the "on" position. But if an electrician comes to do work in your home, or if you are doing any electrical work, even if it is as simple as changing a fuse, you must always disconnect the power by moving the main switch to the "off" position.

CAUTION

You must never open the door of a main electrical switch box. And that means *never!*

If you suspect trouble inside the main switch, call your electrician. Even with a burned-out main fuse and the switch in the "off" position, the electrical contacts are still live and very dangerous.

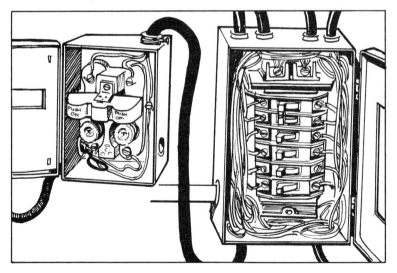

The fuse box (left) has screw-in fuses. The circuit-breaker box (right) requires that you return a switch to the "on" position when it flips off due to a power overload.

Fuses

Inside the main switch box, there is a panelboard that splits the power into circuits that go to the various rooms in your house. Fuses or circuit breakers protect each circuit. If trouble occurs – such as a short circuit or an overload – the fuse blows (burns out) or the circuit breaker trips to the "off" position, and the flow of power to that particular circuit is stopped.

Your fusebox is probably in the basement. It generally requires little maintenance. Proper care is usually as simple as making sure you use the right type and right size of fuse. If you don't, you can overload a circuit and that can lead to a power failure or to a *fire*!

There are a number of warning signals that indicate possible fusebox problems.
• Your fuses burn out repeatedly for no apparent reason, or the circuit breakers repeatedly open automatically.
• You find rust in the fusebox.
• The fusebox becomes discoloured.
• The fusebox becomes overheated.
• Your house lights develop a constant flicker.

These are signals that *must not* be ignored. Call your electrician or electrical contractor. The problem may be solved simply, but this is one of those "better safe than sorry" situations.

To avoid fusebox problems, always remember the following:
• The door or cover of the fusebox should always be kept closed. This will protect children from injury and will prevent dirt from accumulating in the box.
• When going to change a fuse, always have a flashlight with you. Never change a fuse in the dark.
• *Never* change a fuse while standing on a wet floor.
• *Never* change a fuse with the main breaker on.
• Before changing a fuse, turn off the main switch.
• *Always* unplug the appliances on an overloaded circuit before you change the fuse.

- *Never* use a fuse that is larger than that called for. All lighting and general-use circuits are rated at 15 amperes (amps).
- *Never* use a coin or a metal object of any kind to replace a fuse. This eliminates the very protection that a fuse is designed to create. It's the easiest way to start a fire.
- For appliances that use a lot of electricity, use time-delay or dual-element fuses. These are identified by the letters "P" or "D." The "P" fuse is recommended on circuits to appliances that heat but aren't motorized, such as water heaters, baseboard heaters, and ranges. The "D" fuse should be used for large motorized appliances – clothes dryers, furnaces, refrigerators, freezers, and window air conditioners – because they are able to handle power surges that occur normally when the appliance motor is activated.
- Screw in plug-type fuses as tightly as possible (by hand) and check them periodically to ensure that they are screwed in tightly. A loose fuse can overheat.
- If your power is off throughout the entire house, check to see if the power appears to be off in neighbouring houses. If not, the trouble could be in your main switch. Do *not* tackle the job yourself – call your power company.

Electrical Cords and Plugs

Many accidents and injuries associated with electricity are caused by human factors: lack of information, indifference, overconfidence, or foolhardiness. The chances people take with electricity involve common appliances. The main causes of electrical fires are faulty extension cords, carelessly handled appliances, and the misuse of wall plugs.

Extension and replacement cords have, like appliances, changed a good deal over the years. The first cords used with electrical appliances were permanently attached, and the appliances could be used no further from the wall socket than the length of the appliance cord. Then the idea was conceived of making extension cords so that appliances could be used further away from the electrical outlets. Today, not only can you buy extension cords that can handle a variety of appliances at once, but you can also get cords made for specific appliances or types of appliances. Yet, while extension and replacement cords often make life easier for most users, if used improperly they carry a hidden cost in terms of injury and death.

Most victims of electric-cord accidents are children between the ages of six months and four years. A chief cause of these injuries is that water, saliva, and wet diapers are conductors of electricity. Small children often suck and bite on cords, tug at them with their hands and mouths, trip over them, make toys of them, and enjoy playing with them. The results can be serious injuries, disfigurement, and death.

If there are small children in your home, use an extension cord only when it's absolutely necessary. Remember that you must take care of electric cords and plugs just as carefully as you do the appliances they are connected to.

Avoid Trouble

There are a number of other simple rules to prevent electrical catastrophes in the home:

- Never overload a wall socket by adding extension plugs so that a single socket is made to supply electricity for more than a single appliance. These "octopus" connections are one of the greatest of fire hazards. If you feel forced into a situation such as that, it means that you need more outlets installed in your home.
- Make sure that all wall sockets are properly wired and grounded.
- Three-pronged plugs (the ones with the additional round prong that "grounds" the circuit) should always be placed into three-hole wall sockets. Never cut off the third prong because you have an old-fashioned socket. The purpose of these plugs to provide grounding that helps prevent, or minimize, shocks.

CAUTION

The three-hole adapter plug has not been given approval in all communities. Check your local regulations to determine whether you would be using such an adapter legally. If you are allowed to use a properly grounded three-hole adapter to place into your two-hole wall socket, make sure to connect the grounding wire to the screw holding the socket plate.

- Check extension and appliance cords for signs of wear. Don't use a worn or frayed cord.
- Electric cords for lamps, or any other appliances, should never be run under carpets, through doorways, or in any other place in the house that gets extensive wear. Cords are not designed to be walked on. And never place an extension or appliance cord over exposed nails in woodwork.
- If an appliance is exposed to water or other moisture, such as steam, the electrical cord must have a waterproof insulation. Water can damage the normal insulation on an electric cord and thus create a shock hazard.
- Cool your electric iron or other electrical appliances, such as curling irons, before wrapping the extension cord around them when you put them away.
- Never use an appliance or tool that exceeds the electrical rating suggested on your outlet. For example, if the lamp you just bought says to use a 60-watt bulb, do *not* use a 100-watt bulb simply because you want more light.
- Have all your wall outlets covered with safety caps, so that they are covered when not in use. This is especially necessary if you have young children in the house.
- Make sure all plugs fit securely in wall outlets or extension plugs.
- Keep appliance cords or extensions away from radiators or other high heat sources. Heat can damage the insulation on an electric cord and create a shock hazard.

- If you have an appliance plugged into an extension cord semi-permanently, tape the plug in place to prevent children from unplugging it.
- Never use an extension cord that is longer than it has to be. Your hardware store will sell you a holder in which you can safely wrap the unneeded length of wire so that your extension will not act as a trip-over hazard.
- Inspect both the cord and the plug on all your appliances. If they are worn, they could cause a fire, or create a short-circuit, or give you a shock. If they are worn or damaged, replace them and discard the worn ones.
- Never pull the plug from the socket by the cord. That will only wear the cord quickly, and the result can be a shock hazard.
- Extension cords should never be used as permanent wiring.

Above all, if a fire should start due to faulty wiring or any other electrical cause, never, *never*, **never** use water to try to extinguish the flames. There is a serious shock hazard in doing so.

Your Appliances and Their Use

Today, electrical appliances, if used safely and with care, make life easier and relieve drudgery. Before buying an electrical appliance, make sure it has a seal of certification. This might be the CSA seal (the certification mark of the Canadian Standards Association) or the UL seal (the Underwriters Laboratory in the United States). Next, *before* you use your appliance, read the accompanying literature. Follow the manufacturer's instructions and keep them handy so that you can keep yourself informed about operation and care.

The following are a few general rules for using household appliances:
- Disconnect an appliance before cleaning it.
- Never touch a plugged-in appliance if your hands are damp.
- If an appliance sparks, overheats, or stalls, pull the plug and have it checked by the dealer or the appliance service centre.

- Never pry toast out of the toaster with a fork or knife unless you unplug it first.
- Electrical appliances of any kind – radios, hair dryers, curling irons, shavers – are a hazard near water. Even if your hands are damp, or you're standing on a wet floor or a wet bathmat, you could get a serious shock or other injury.

Don't Do It to Yourself

Do-it-yourself has been popular for the past several decades. And in all that time, the number of accidents suffered by do-it-yourselfers has led safety experts to warn against the dangers of doing it *to* yourself.

Are you installing an antenna for your CB, TV, or other communications system? Make sure it is installed well away from power lines. A good formula is to measure the height of the antenna, add ten feet, and then install the antenna that distance away from any power line so that you can feel somewhat safe. If you're putting up a twenty-foot antenna, install it at least thirty feet from the nearest power line. And while you're getting up on the roof, or wherever, to start your installation, make sure your ladder doesn't touch that power line.

Are you doing some long-range gardening? Planting trees so that you can have shade for your back patio in five or six years? Or getting a willow so that the swampy part of your backyard will be soaked up by the ever-thirsty tree? Look up! Are there power lines above where the tree will be growing? No problem today, but when that tree starts to reach full height then the problems will begin.

And if you already have a tree or trees growing into power lines, do *not* attempt to prune them yourself. Nor should you fell the tree yourself. If a large branch, or the tree, falls on a line, it could be fatal for you. Call your power company and tell them about the problem.

When you are working near power lines (painting the house, repairing the roof or the chimney) don't touch or even come close to touching those lines – yourself or with your equipment. Touching even the equipment could cause serious injury.

And if you're digging, first call both your local power company and your telephone company. Let them locate underground power and phone lines for you. To cut through a power line is dangerous. And cutting through either a power or a phone line could black out an entire area.

When your home was built, the entire electrical installation was inspected to ensure that it measured up to the electrical safety code of your community. If you add to your wiring, make sure that you have it inspected.

Teaching Your Children

Throughout this book we stress the need for making sure your children are aware of the dangers around the home. Because children make use of electrical appliances with ease – and often without warning – warn them ahead of time:

• Never touch a downed wire. Even if it appears dead, touching it could be fatal.
• Never keep electric clocks, electric barbecues, electric radios, or TVs near a swimming pool.
• Never stick fingers or playthings into wall outlets.

CAUTION

Keep electric heaters and fans away from curious youngsters, and never leave irons, toasters, or small appliances within the reach of youngsters who are unattended.

Electrical Emergencies

You have already learned something about handling electrical fires from the first chapter of this book. You are aware that you must never use water on a fire that has been generated by an electrical source. You cannot use water on electrical equipment or wires, because water is a good conductor of electricity and you could get a severe shock.

If an electrically based fire starts, make sure *you are not grounded* and use a non-conductor to try to unplug the equipment. Use a dry-chemical electrical fire extinguisher, or baking soda, to put out the fire. (See chart on page 24.)

If someone inside your home receives a shock from a faulty appliance and is still in contact with it: 1. *Don't* touch the appliance. 2. *Don't* touch the victim. 3. Make sure you are not grounded, and use a non-conductor to unplug it from the wall socket (see pages 124-126). 4. Once the victim is free from the faulty appliance or power line, begin first aid. Have someone else call for an ambulance; don't leave the victim unattended.

If the victim is unconscious or breathing erratically, use artificial respiration immediately. Every second counts.

Power Failures

Most power systems today are very reliable, but power outages are possible. Sometimes the failure can be widespread and long-lasting.

The possible causes of a power failure are many. Weather is a common cause. Ice or snow on power lines can break them. Wind can blow down power lines. Accidents – such as a car hitting a power pole, or a construction crew cutting a power line – can cause a power failure in your home.

If the power is off in the homes or apartments around you, then it is a break in the system and the power company crews will repair it. If the failure blacks out your entire house, but only your house, then it could be your main switch. Do not attempt to repair it yourself. Call your power company.

Most power companies maintain a storm-watch system to prepare themselves as far in advance as possible for emergencies. But should a major storm disrupt service in your area, there are some things you should do to lessen the inconvenience of being without power.

WATER. If there is sufficient warning before a storm, fill your bathtub and spare containers with water because the water-pumping system in your community or in your home could be affected by a power failure. Store as much water as you can for drinking, cooking, and washing. Toilets can be flushed by pouring a bucket of water in the bowl.

FOOD. Before the storm hits, turn the controls on your refrigerator and freezer to the coldest possible setting. Food will stay frozen between 36 and 48 hours in a fully loaded freezer if you keep the door closed. Ice cream is an exception and should be discarded.

If the freezer is only half-full, the food will generally keep for 24 hours. A freezer full of meat generally keeps frozen longer than a freezer full of baked goods. Meat that has ice crystals remaining in it may be refrozen. Most bakery goods can be refrozen.

Most refrigerator food will keep for 24 hours. Dairy products such as milk, cream, sour cream, yogurt, and cottage cheese should be discarded after six to eight hours. So think about what you want *before* you open the refrigerator door; in that way no more cold air than necessary can escape.

Return refrigerator or freezer controls to their normal settings when service is restored.

If the storm hits during the winter, you can prolong the time that food will not spoil by storing it in a cold place outside your home, such as an unheated garage or tool shed.

RADIOS AND FLASHLIGHTS. Transistor radios and flashlights supplied with fresh batteries should be in every home. Candles should be used carefully and should be kept out of drafts, and out of the reach of children.

Radio stations will broadcast timely progress reports on efforts to restore service.

APPLIANCES. Disconnect or shut off any appliances that will go on automatically when power is restored. Such appliances include furnaces, air conditioners, water heaters, refrigerators, freezers, and water pumps.

Make sure electric space heaters, washers, dryers, and television sets are shut off. If a number of appliances come on at once, they may overload the electric circuits and cause a power failure in your home. Also, appliances may begin operating when you are away or asleep.

A single lamp may be left turned on to alert you that power has been restored. And when service is restored, your appliances should be turned on one at a time.

COOKING. During an emergency, a camp stove, your fireplace, or a can of Sterno (placed in a holder on a flame-proof surface) can be used for cooking. Propane-burning camp stoves should be used only with proper ventilation.

Freeze-dried or dehydrated foods of the kind used by campers and backpackers can be prepared with a minimum of heat.

CAUTION

Never use a barbecue indoors; charcoal emits carbon monoxide, which can kill by asphyxiation.

FISHTANKS. If you have fish in a tank, a small bicycle pump can supply air to them during a power failure.

DOWNED WIRES. If you should see downed wires around your home, do not attempt to touch them or move them. Treat them as if they are "live." It is especially important to keep children away from them. Report downed wires to the police or to your electric power company.

Winter Power Failures

An extended power failure during the winter months, and subsequent loss of heating, can result in cold, damp homes, severe living conditions, as well as damage to walls, floors, and plumbing.

The consequences of power and heating failure in subfreezing weather can be reduced in two ways: protect your home against frost damage if you should leave for a vacation;

and have an emergency standby heating system that will permit continued occupancy throughout an emergency.

Advance Precautions

Winter power failures are one of the common emergencies that anyone can be prepared for. The following six suggestions will help:

• If you have a fireplace, keep a good supply of fuel on hand.

• Install a standby stove or heater that does not require electricity, and make sure it is vented. One way of doing this is by connecting it to an unused flue. Use only fuel-burning heaters that are appropriately certified.

• If the standby heating unit will use the normal house oil or gas supply, have it connected with shut-off valves by a competent serviceman from the fuel supplier.

• Have flashlights, lanterns, candles, and matches, or other emergency lighting devices stored in a handy place. (See "Emergency Cupboard" on page 41.)

• Check with your local supply authority before arranging for installation of emergency generators for furnaces, appliances, or lighting.

• Have a battery-powered radio and spare batteries to keep you informed. Many radio stations can operate using emergency power.

Don't Panic

Remember that even in very cold weather, a house with doors and windows closed will not become unendurable for several hours. If you have a standby heating unit, turn it on before the house gets too cold. If the unit must be vented to the same chimney flue as the furnace, switch the furnace off before disconnecting the furnace flue.

A house can be damaged by low temperatures, but the major threat is to the plumbing system. If a standby heating system is used, check to see that no part of the plumbing system can freeze. If all or part of a house must be abandoned, protect it by taking the following precautions:

1. Turn off the main electric switch.
2. Turn off the water main where it enters the house. Protect the valve, inlet pipe, and meter or pump with blankets or insulating material.
3. Open all water taps in the house slightly, drain the water heater, and flush toilets until they are empty of water.
4. Check the operating manual that came with your dishwasher, washing machine, etc., for draining or frost protection instructions.
5. Horizontal water supply lines, which might not drain when valves are open, should be blown out with a tire pump.

Listen to a battery-operated or car radio for more detailed instructions. If your local broadcast station is off the air, try tuning to others in the area.

After the power returns, switch on the main switch. Then replace the furnace flue (if it was removed) and turn off the fuel to the standby heating unit. Turn on the water supply, closing lowest valves first to allow air to escape from the upper taps.

Make sure the hot water heater is filled with water before turning on the power. If necessary, rinse out the dishwasher and washing machine.

Warm the house slightly above normal temperature for a few hours to allow it to dry thoroughly.

Emergency Cupboard

You should have a cupboard stocked with such emergency items as batteries, matches, flashlights, candles and holders, and/or a portable battery lamp.

A fondue pot with a fuel supply can be used for heating food.

It is also a good idea to have a transistor radio and a non-electric alarm clock.

When Power Resumes

1. Check to see that the freezer and refrigerator are working, and which of the foods can be refrozen, if defrosting has occurred.

2. Reset clocks and check automatic timers and alarms.
3. Plug in only the most essential appliances; waiting ten to fifteen minutes before reconnecting everything gives the electrical system time to stabilize.
4. Replace all emergency supplies in the emergency cupboard.

CHAPTER **3**

Protecting Your Home Against Intruders

A RESIDENTIAL BURGLARY occurs every three and a half minutes in Canada. Since the beginning of the 1980s, the number of cases of breaking and entering reported to the police has increased by about 25 per cent. The risk of a break-in on some city streets is more than one in eight houses.

The most obvious way to protect against such criminal acts would be to have a burglar-proof house built. The next best – and more reasonable – approach is to evaluate your living quarters, determine its weak points, and prepare to create as burglar-proof a home for yourself as possible.

When we talk of burglary, we refer to breaking and entering. There is no personal threat involved. When your home is broken into while you're out, that's a burglary. But you need not be out; you could be asleep or in some other part of the house or on the grounds when the break-in takes place.

While the victims naturally decry the fact that they have had their personal rights violated, the truth is that too often the victim has left himself open to that violation. The break-in is often facilitated by unlocked doors and windows. Or people leave on vacation paying no attention to the fact that there are obvious signs that no one is at home.

There are countless other ways in which people "give away" clues to criminals. For example, a newspaper obituary notice will list the time and place of the funeral services. There is every expectation that all members of the deceased's household will attend the services. Burglars know this and regularly read the obituaries to find temporarily empty homes. Or, you retire at night and turn off all the lights. Yet lights – especially those outdoors – are the major enemy of the burglar. Perhaps you leave town for several weeks and have your telephone disconnected. A temporary disconnection may be an indication that you haven't paid your bill – or that you are out of town. Finally, you normally leave your draperies open, but when leaving town for a few days you draw them.

There are ways to combat these give-away situations:

- While the funeral service is going on, arrange for someone to house-sit.
- Leave some lights on every night, preferably outside lights at the front, side, and back doors.
- Do not disconnect your telephone when you take a trip; the cost of a few weeks' service is cheap compared to the loss that can occur if a would-be burglar tries to call and discovers you are not at home. To combat the possibility that a would-be burglar might hear your phone ringing unanswered, turn the bell down as far as it will go while you're away.
- If you normally draw the draperies at night but leave them open during the day, arrange for a neighbour to come in and do that while you are away.

To protect your home, look at the areas of ingress. How is a burglar going to get in? The most obvious point of entry to any home is the door. If it is unlocked, you have made it too easy for the criminal. Yet this is the way most illegal entries are made. Many families never trouble to lock their front doors – some even leave the door unlocked after they've gone to bed. And if there are young children in the house, it is very tempting to leave the door unlocked so that the youngsters can get in and out easily throughout the day.

Problem Doors

Your first line of defence in the house is a locked door. That doesn't guarantee protection. There are a number of ways in which a determined burglar can get around a locked door. For example:

- Some types of locks can be picked easily or actually removed from the door from outside the house.
- A door that does not fit the door frame tightly can be pried open.
- Doors that open to the outside have hinges on the outside. All a determined criminal has to do is remove the hinges and lift the door out of its frame.
- Doors with glass windows, or even decorative wood panels, are susceptible to being broken through. Then the burglar reaches in to unlock the door.

Lock Your Doors

So how do you protect a door, now that you have been made aware that its physical presence is not necessarily a deterrent to entry? It is essential that the door be made of a sturdy material. The best door is made of metal. Second best is a solid wood door. If, however, you prefer a door with glass or wood panels – the kind that is more susceptible to break-in – then your protection has to come from the inside: the lock.

There are a variety of locking devices that your locksmith can install for you. These include:

THE DEAD-BOLT. This is the best type of lock in any situation. This lock has a square-faced hardened-steel bolt (in contrast to the triangular shape of the common type that locks itself as the door closes) that is activated from the inside by a second turn of the key. There are several variations of this excellent deterrent to entry through the door. A dead-bold lock can be used independently, or can be made a supplementary lock to any other you have on your doors.

THE DOUBLE-CYLINDER LOCK. This is the second-best type to have. This requires a key to open it from both the outside and the inside. True, it isn't as convenient as other kinds of locks – and with young children in the house it could be a nuisance – but it is most effective on decoratively panelled doors.

There is one serious drawback to a double-cylinder lock. In case of fire, it can delay your getting out of the house. So make sure that there is a key to the inside lock in a convenient place – and that everyone who lives there knows where it is. Also, check with your fire department for local rules and regulations in this regard.

PUSHBUTTON COMBINATION LOCKS. These can't be opened by a burglar with a picklock (a device that fits into the key slot and can be adjusted to manipulate the tumblers into an "open" position). The problem with this type of lock is that a determined thief can "read" the combination as you manipulate your lock, and do so from a reasonable distance. It is a better lock to use on an inside door if you have a security situation.

PICKPROOF LOCKS. Various types are available, but they are expensive and only if you have items of exceedingly great value in your home might it be worth the expense of such an installation.

THE NIGHT LATCH. These were common for many years, but they do not offer much protection. This is the kind of lock you often see being opened with ease – if you watch TV crime shows – by using a plastic credit card.

THE LOCK-IN-THE-KNOB. This device is commonly used in apartment houses. It is a weak protection because it can be easily pried loose and has proven to be the entry point for many burglaries.

CHAIN LOCKS. These can be made more effective if mounted with bolts or even long screws, but even then there is a limit to their protective value. Usually a good kick will pull them free from the wall. And the chain itself is always susceptible to a bolt cutter or hacksaw. However, the addition of a chain lock to your other locking device might be useful for several reasons. It will show a burglar, if he manages to get the door unlocked, that someone is at home, and he'll leave. (On the other hand, if he gets into the house and then puts the chain lock on, he'll be warned if anyone comes home and tries to get in.) And if you have a solid front door, without a peephole, it permits you to open the door partially to determine who a "visitor" is.

As we noted earlier, exterior doors hinged on the outside will provide burglars with easy access to your home. They have only to remove the hinge pins and lift the door out of its frame. This situation can be corrected in three ways: have the door removed and hinges remounted on the inside of the frame so the door swings inward; install a set of non-removable hinge pins; or install a locking pin in each of the existing hinge plates as follows:

- Remove the centre screw from each plate of both the top and bottom hinges of the door.
- Insert "headless" screws or bolts into the door jamb through the holes in the hinge plates, leaving one-half inch protruding.
- Drill three-quarter-inch holes through the opposing hinge plates into the door.

Once this is done, the pins in the door jamb will penetrate the holes in the door. The door will then be held in position even if the hinge pins are removed.

Locking a sliding patio door is a different problem altogether. The usual lock may deter an intruder, but then a glass-cutter is all that is needed to get through the door, or at least to get at the lock. Vertical bolts that fit into holes at floor and ceiling levels of the door can hold it firmly in place when locked. Some people cut a broom handle to fit the track in which the door slides, so that even if the lock is forced the panel cannot slide open. The only avenue left for the would-be burglar then is to break the glass. Therefore, shatter-proof panes are needed to make the patio door all but impenetrable.

What if you lose your door keys? A lot will depend on whether you keep your keys separate from any identification. If you don't, then anyone who finds them and has a mind to burglarize your home has an easy way in. If you lose your keys, have a locksmith realign the inner works – the pins – and cut new keys for you.

Finally, having glass panels or a peephole in the door is valuable in that you can see who is ringing your doorbell, and if it's someone you don't know and might be wary of, you can open with care. This is where a chain lock can be helpful. A second precaution, if you feel you need it, is to have a wedge-shaped rubber doorstop to slip beneath the door. This provides added assistance to the chain lock and could give you sufficient time, while the would-be intruder recoils from the shock of the door not budging, to slam the door shut and call for help.

Protect Your Windows

Windows provide little security. Therefore, the first rule of window protection is to evaluate all the windows in your home. Those that are not necessary for ventilation purposes should be made permanently secure. You may find that some of your windows were "frozen" shut the last time the house was painted. This is an inexpensive method of permanently securing windows not needed for ventilation.

As a general rule, a would-be burglar will not break a window. There are two sensible reasons for this from the intruder's point of view. First, a shattering window makes considerable noise, and attention is the last thing the housebreaker wants to arouse. Second, a broken window may expose him to sharp edges and injury, which he also wants to avoid.

This does not mean, however, that the burglar will not use a glass cutter to remove a section of the window pane in order to reach the window lock – especially the butterfly-type locks that most people have on their windows. This is the kind of lock found on windows that slide up and down, otherwise known as double-hung windows. If the window is loose fitting, the butterfly lock can be opened easily be slipping a knife blade, or other thin strip of metal, through the crack separating the frames.

Windows needed for ventilation can be protected in a variety of ways. A heavy nail or screw can be driven into the window track at a spot that will prevent the window from being raised high enough for anyone to crawl through. But don't limit this method to only one side of the window. Place your "stoppers" in both tracks. Key-operated locks are another effective method, especially for windows on the first floor of your house. Finally, bars or window guards are excellent deterrents – but these also prevent getting out of the house through a window in case of fire or other emergency.

Check the putty around your window panes yearly – especially if you haven't had the interior of the house painted during the past year. Putty dries out and makes removal of a window pane far easier than you would like. If the painter didn't replace the putty the last time he painted your house, do it yourself. And next time, insist that he do it.

Casement windows that are opened with a crank-like appliance from the inside provide more protection than the double-hung variety.

Ground-floor windows, obviously, provide a greater risk than those in the upper floor or floors of your house. But check the upper storeys: are the windows near balconies, fire escapes, trees, or even the roof? Is a next-door neighbour close enough that access to an upper-floor window could be gained from the house next door? If any one of these possibilities exists, then you must treat the windows upstairs with as much care as those on the ground floor.

Window security checks should include basement and storeroom windows, ventilation exhausts, coal chutes, storm cellars, attics, and any other space that can provide access to your home. And basement windows hidden by bushes or trees provide burglars with an ideal place to work unobserved. Such windows can be replaced with plexiglass or Lexan, or reinforced with decorative security bars. Seldom-used basement windows should be permanently secured.

Finally, if you have window air-conditioners, make sure that they cannot be removed easily from the outside. This may entail securing them to the window and the window frame with screws or by placing a bar across the face of the unit that is securely attached to the walls inside the house.

Safety from the Inside

An alarm system is the best way to provide protection from within your house. There are a number of kinds. Some will detect intruders only. Some will also detect fires. And the kind that seems most useful is the one that can be activated by someone in the house in the event of any emergency.

Smoke detectors have been discussed in the first chapter of this book. along with this essential alarm system you should consider an intruder-alarm device. Seek help from an expert in the field to determine what might work best in your home. The best-known types of intrusion detection devices are:

METALLIC TAPE. This is placed on all window surfaces and works on the principle that if the window is broken, so is the tape. This interrupts an electric current and sounds the alarm. Its weakness is that an intruder can use a glass cutter and leave the tape undisturbed.

PRESSURE DETECTORS. These look something like doormats. If an intruder steps on the mat, electrical contacts are brought together and the alarm is sounded.

PHOTOELECTRIC DETECTORS. The intruder activates this device by interrupting a beam of light, but it can be circumvented by ducking under the beam or stepping around or over it. To eliminate that problem, some of these devices utilize infrared beams that cannot be seen by the naked eye.

MAGNETIC SWITCHES. This device is operated by a magnet that holds one of the contacts of a switch away from the other. The magnet is attached to the door, the switch to the frame. When the door is opened, the magnet no longer holds the contact in place and an alarm is sounded.

SOUND-WAVE SENSORS. Sound waves too high to be heard by the human ear are transmitted to fill a room. When an intruder enters, the pattern of the waves is altered and an alarm sounds.

ELECTROMAGNETIC-WAVE DETECTORS. Similar to the above, these devices can work beyond one room.

Above all, don't "advertise" the fact that you have any protective devices working to protect your home. The fewer outsiders who know what system you use for intruder-protection, the better your system can operate.

Safety on the Outside

High walls, dead-end driveways, and heavy shrubbery provide protective cover for intruders. When we plan the aesthetic view of our homes from the outside, we often forget that we may be sacrificing security. High walls and other such barriers should be lit at night. Shrubbery should be trimmed so that maximum visibility exists.

If you let the shrubs outside your home grow high enough to conceal an intruder, by day or by night, you are asking for trouble. The same applies to any type of concealment: a cord of wood neatly stacked for use in your fireplace next winter; empty cartons from new appliances you just installed, piled to await the refuse collection later in the week; the large pile of tree limbs you pruned last weekend and have left for the garbage collector to pick up.

Fencing your property is a fine idea, but building a fence that protects you from the view of passersby protects intruders from being seen by passersby or neighbours. If you want a fence or a hedge around your house, don't make it so high that it works against you as well as for you.

Your garage is another means of access to your home, especially if there is an entry from the garage to the house. In some communities, this is illegal for fire-protection reasons and that regulation serves a double purpose: it eliminates an easy way into your home.

If there is entry to the house from the garage, then garage doors should be locked at all times. Automatic door-opening devices will make life a little easier for you in this circumstance – and while the radio-operated door-openers are most convenient, they can often be triggered by a transmitter in a passing automobile or even one on an airplane overhead. The preferable type is key-operated by means of a lock-trigger that is set in a stanchion on the driver's side of the driveway near the garage doors.

Whether you have automatic doors or not for your garage, avoid stacking anything or keeping bulky items in the garage in a way that could provide a hiding place for an intruder.

Padlocks should be used for the back or side door of your garage, as well as for the doors to storm cellars, tool sheds, and other small buildings on your property. And padlocks are less than useful if the hasps and hinges are poor quality. If hinges are exposed, treat them as suggested above for exposed front-door hinges.

Safety While You're Away

When you are going away for any length of time, and no one will be at home, take specific precautions to prevent leaving the house susceptible to break-in.

• Discontinue mail and newspaper delivery if you can't arrange with a neighbour to visit your house at the appropriate times to take in the papers and mail. If you cancel, however, you could be "signalling" that you are away, so cancellation should be done as a last resort.

• Make sure that all possible entrances to your home are secured.

- Tell your neighbours that you are going to be away, and for how long. Leave a key with a neighbour you trust.
- Many police forces like to know if your home is vacant, particularly if you have an alarm system. Let the police know if you will be having a neighbour come in from time to time.
- Use timer switches for lights and a radio so that lights go on and off at times that are normal for your household activities. A random switch is useful in that it makes the activity of the lights less obviously programmed.
- Arrange to keep your lawn cut or to have the snow removed so that everything looks normal around the house. If snow can't be shovelled immediately, arrange with the neighbour to have footprints on your walkway until the shovelling is done. Nothing is as much a giveaway to an empty house in winter as pristine snow.
- If you're going to be away for some time, arrange with a neighbour to put out some of his trash or garbage at your house so that you have a pick-up done, too.
- If you normally leave your draperies open, don't close them when you go away. If you close them at night and leave them open during the day, try to get a neighbour to come in daily to rearrange them that way; otherwise leave them open.

Apartment Security

While the building superintendent or the police seem safe to fall back on if you're an apartment dweller, the security of the apartment building you live in is only as effective as you make it.

The following nine steps will help you keep your apartment secure:
- When the buzzer rings, check the identity of the person or persons seeking entrance before you release the spring latch on the lobby door.
- Unknown or suspicious persons seeking entrance to the building should be referred to the superintendent.

- Notify the superintendent when your apartment will be vacant for any length of time.
- Make arrangements with a neighbour or the superintendent to receive deliveries. Do not leave notes on the lobby callboard.
- Do not identify yourself on the callboard as a female living alone. First initials will identify you; e.g., S.D. Jones.
- When moving into a new apartment, have the lock cylinder changed. Before changing or replacing locks in your apartment, check with the superintendent. Permission is usually required.
- Your apartment door should be equipped with good-quality deadbolt locks. Install a wide-angle door viewer.
- Secure sliding doors on the balcony with "jimmy bars," or cut a broom stick to place in the bottom track, making sure it fits snugly.
- Good-quality locks should be placed on all windows, especially those opening onto balconies or rooftops.

CHAPTER 4

Storms: Hurricanes and Tornadoes

CHANCES ARE YOU HAVE often had to deal with the effects of storms. You probably know some of the problems that storms can cause. But have you ever wondered what you would do if your community were struck by a severe storm, possible even a tornado or a hurricane? The heavy precipitation, strong winds, and lightning that accompany such a storm can damage property and endanger lives. It is essential, therefore, that you know what types of storms could occur in your area and at what time of the year they are likely to strike.

The appropriate government agencies and the broadcast media co-operate to provide weather warnings. If you are listening to radio (or are watching television) you will be warned when a storm is approaching your area. The next step is to know what you can do to protect your family and your home.

Things To Do Now

Storms strike quickly. Therefore, some things cannot be left until the warnings are issued. You must think about them now.

PREPARE YOUR EMERGENCY PACK. This should include an emergency food supply as well as extra clothing, blankets, medication, and first-aid items. Your battery-powered radio and spare batteries should be included, too – they might be the only link you'll have with the outside world. You might want to include tools for making emergency repairs, as well as flashlights, lanterns, or other emergency lighting.

CHOOSE YOUR SHELTER. Your basement, a storm cellar or fall-out shelter, or a spot beneath a staircase or underneath sturdy furniture on the ground floor in the centre of the building away from outside walls and windows are all good places to ride out storms. If you are planning home improvements in the near future, you might want to consider strengthening an interior room against storm winds.

REDUCE THE HAZARDS. Trim dead or rotting branches and cut down dead trees to reduce the danger of limbs falling on your home. Check the landscaping, and be extra mindful of the drainage around your house.

PROTECT AGAINST FLOODING. High winds can cause unusually high waves and tides. Heavy rains associated with hurricanes and other windstorms can lead to sudden or flash flooding in low-lying and coastal areas. (See Chapter Five.)

CHOOSE A RENDEZVOUS. When a severe storm strikes, you might be separated from members of your family who are at home, at work, or at school. Avoid unnecessary worry and travel by arranging now to have a family meeting-place or system of communication after a storm to ensure that no one is lost or in need of help.

ENSURE MOBILITY AFTERWARDS. Always have a fairly full tank of gasoline in your car. Filling station pumps may not operate for several days after a storm.

In the Storm Season

When a severe storm threatens:
• Keep your local radio or television station turned on so that you can hear warnings and advice as soon as they are broadcast. Keep your battery-powered radio handy – the electrical power may fail.

- If you have the time, board up the windows with securely fastened lumber or close storm shutters. You can also use tape to strengthen windows.
- Use strong bracing to make outside doors secure. But when the storm begins, open doors and windows slightly *on the side of the house away from the storm* to help equalize pressure and thus reduce the hazard of implosion. Remember to stay away from doors and windows to avoid flying glass and debris.
- Secure anything that might be blown around or torn loose, both indoors and out. Flying objects such as garbage cans and lawn furniture can damage property and injure people. Storing belongings indoors can also protect against damage from hail.
- Avoid travelling. You don't want to be caught without shelter. Protect your automobile by slightly lowering windows and setting brakes. If your garage is sturdy, store cars there.
- If you are advised by officials to evacuate, do so. But if you live on the waterfront, don't go by boat! Take your emergency kit and supplies with you. You will also need flashlights and batteries, infant-care supplies, and personal documents and identification for each family member. Before you leave, shut off electricity to reduce fire hazard.
- If a storm reaches severe proportions, go to your shelter spot. Take your emergency kit with you.
- If a storm or tornado catches you outdoors, take shelter immediately. As a last resort, lie flat in a ditch, excavation, or culvert.

Above all, *keep calm*. You'll be more able to cope with emergencies if you don't panic.

After the Storm

Listen to your radio for information and instructions after the storm passes. And follow those instructions.

Give first aid to injured or trapped persons and/or get help if necessary. But unless you are qualified, or are requested to help, stay away from damaged areas. Particularly stay away from loose or dangling electrical wiring. Report them to authorities. Also report broken sewer or water mains.

Lightning and downed power lines can cause fires. Know how to fight small fires. (See Chapter One.) Contact the fire department. Be alert to prevent fires; remember, broken water mains may cause lowered water pressure and fire-fighting will be impaired.

Don't use your car unless it is extremely important. Nor should you use your telephone except in extreme emergencies.

If your power has been off for several hours, check freezers and refrigerators for spoiling food. (See Chapter Two.) Water may also be contaminated after a storm so purify your drinking and cooking water by boiling or adding purification tablets or chlorinating. (See Chapter Five.)

Lightning

More people are killed by lightning throughout the year than by the other effects of violent storms. Lightning is an electrical discharge resulting from the build-up of static electricity between clouds and the ground, or between clouds themselves. It is present in all thunderstorms and even more frequently in severe ones.

To estimate the distance of a lightning bolt – and thereby determine whether you need to take shelter because the lightning is nearby – count the number of seconds between the flash you see and the thunderclap you hear. Every second indicates a distance of 300 metres (about 1,000 feet), and if there is a time lapse of less than five seconds between flash and clap, take shelter. The lightning is too close for safety.

When there is lightning activity, don't go outdoors unless it is absolutely necessary. And while indoors, keep away from doors, windows, fireplaces, radiators, stoves, metal pipes, sinks, or appliances that will conduct electricity.

During a severe thunderstorm it may be wise to disconnect televisions and radios; and don't handle electrical appliances or telephones.

If you have been caught outdoors, seek shelter in a building, cave, or depressed area. If you are in the water – swimming or in a small boat – get back to shore immediately. Keep away from wire or metal fences and telephone lines or power lines. Don't use any equipment such as lawn mowers, golf carts, tractors, bicycles, or motorcycles. Get off and away from them. Avoid using shovels, golf clubs, clotheslines, etc., and try not to be the tallest object in the area.

If you're caught in the open, kneel with your feet close together and lower your head. Do not lie flat, and don't take shelter under a tree or on a hilltop.

If you're in a car, stay there. You have the best protection. However, if you've stopped the car near a tree, pull away lest it fall on you.

Tornadoes

Tornadoes, or "twisters," are violent windstorms characterized by a twisting funnel-shaped cloud that forms at the base of a cloud bank and points toward the ground. Tornadoes usually occur in conjunction with severe thunderstorms and are accompanied by lightning and sometimes heavy rain or hail. Their destructive force comes from the extremely high winds – 150 kilometres (100 miles) an hour and higher – and very low air pressure, which combine to form a tornado.

They strike suddenly, and their loud roaring noise will alert you that one is coming. They move 50 to 70 km/hour (30 to 50 mph) and normally touch ground for less than twenty seconds. If you live in an area that is tornado-prone, keep your battery-operated radio playing during thunderstorms and listen for severe weather warnings. Above all, be prepared because tornadoes strike very quickly.

• Choose a shelter in advance. If you spot a tornado, you probably won't have time to hunt for shelter. Know the best shelter space in your home, in addition to knowing where to seek shelter in your office, school, or workplace.

- Upper floors in a building are unsafe. However, if there is no time to descend, a closet or a small room with stout walls or an inside hallway will give some protection against flying debris. Otherwise, get under a piece of heavy furniture or a tipped-over upholstered couch or chair in the centre part of the room.
- If you don't have a basement, an inner hallway or small inner room away from windows makes the best shelter.
- Avoid large halls, arenas, cafeterias, etc.; their roofs are more likely to collapse.
- Get as close to the ground as you can. Crouch or lie flat on the floor underneath heavy furniture, or under a tipped-over sofa or upholstered chair. Protect your head from debris.
- If you are caught outdoors, hang onto a tree or a stout bush to try to prevent the strong winds from blowing you away.
- If you are driving and spot a tornado heading toward you, try to drive away from its path at a right angle. If you cannot escape the tornado, get out of the car immediately – the car might roll over or be blown through the air. Seek shelter, or lie flat in a depression such as a ditch or a ravine. If there is no shelter close by, get under the car to protect yourself from flying debris.

Blizzards

Treat these severe winters storms with respect. Their high winds, extremely low temperatures, and heavy snowfall can endanger lives in minutes.

- If blizzard or heavy snowsquall warnings are broadcast several days beforehand, make sure you have sufficient heating fuel. Trucks may not be able to get through during a storm.
- Do not go outdoors during a blizzard. Be prepared to wait out the storm indoors.
- Ice and freezing rain can cause power lines to break. Know how to protect yourself and your home in periods of extreme cold. (See Chapters Two and Ten.)

Hurricanes

The violent tropical storms that are all too common in the southern United States can sometimes reach into parts of Canada. Hurricanes cause more widespread damage than tornadoes. By the time a hurricane reaches Canada, heavy rain and flooding are usually greater hazards than the strong winds.

Hurricanes move slowly and an affected community can be battered for hours in such a storm. When they are around coastal areas, they can cause tidal waves or storm surges. Most people killed in hurricanes are caught in these floodwaters.

If the storm suddenly abates, be careful. It may be the "eye" of the storm passing and this will provide a lull of up to a half-hour. Remain in a safe place. Make emergency repairs only if essential.

REMEMBER: when the eye has passed the wind will return suddenly from the opposite direction, with probably even greater force.

When the Storm Is Over

Homes and furnishings damaged as a result of any storm or storm-related disaster need prompt clean-up action.

- Before entering a damaged building, be sure that it is not about to collapse.
- Turn off gas at the meter or tank and let the house air for several minutes to remove foul odors or escaped gas.
- Do not smoke or use open flames until you are sure that it is safe to do so.
- Do not turn on an electrical system; it may have become short-circuited. After dark, use a flashlight to avoid igniting escaped gas.
- Watch out for holes in the floor or loose boards with exposed nails.

Damage from high winds can be extremely great. Tornadoes may demolish some buildings and move others almost intact for some distance from their foundations. Before entering or cleaning a tornado-damaged building, be sure that the walls, ceiling, and roof are in place and that the structure rests firmly on the foundation. Look out for glass and broken power lines.

Of course, flood damage will be far greater than wind damage if a flood has occurred as a result of the storm. The following chapter, concerning floods and flood damage, goes into full details on cleaning up after a flood.

CHAPTER 5

Floods: Survival and Cleaning Up

FLOOD THREATS CAN usually be forecast by constant evaluation of rising water tables resulting from heavy rain, surveys of snow conditions in river drainage basins, meteorological observations and forecasts. Advance warning about floods developing in one or any of these ways is usually available.

On the other hand, in some places there exists the possibility of flash flooding, or sudden flooding, in which warning time is extremely limited. Such flash flooding can result from other causes. Earthquakes, tidal waves, hurricanes, violent storms, or bursting dams can bring floods as devastating as natural overflow of water basins.

Whatever the source of the floodwaters, however, the most reliable information on what is happening in the affected areas – as well as those areas likely to be affected – will come from local government authorities.

Radio and television are usually the fastest means of learning what actions are recommended to take to limit or to prevent disaster. Detailed instructions by municipal or provincial authorities will be designed to meet immediate needs.

Should a Flood Threaten

There are three major areas of concern to you in the event of flood. These are electricity, your heating equipment, and water contamination.

ELECTRICITY. Immediately shut off the power in premises that are in imminent danger of flooding. You have already learned in Chapter Two that water is a conductor of electricity, so you know that the two certainly do not mix.

However, don't attempt to shut off the power if the main switch is in a location that has already been flooded. If conditions are wet around the switch box, stand on a dry board and use a dry stick to turn the switch off. Later in this chapter you will be told how to go about preparing to use electrical equipment after the flood.

HEATING EQUIPMENT. Special precautions should be taken to safeguard or minimize damage to electrical, natural gas, or propane heating equipment. If warning time permits, consult your supplier for steps to be taken. If your heating equipment has been flooded, do not attempt to put it back into service until you have read about the problems of doing so, which are discussed later in this chapter.

WATER CONTAMINATION. If you suspect that your drinking water has been contaminated, purify it before drinking. You will have no trouble easily sensing such contamination; the taste, colour, or odour of the water will not be normal. Purification can be done by boiling the water for at least 10 minutes or chlorinating it with a bleaching compound. How to do this is described later in this chapter.

General Precautions

There are a number of precautions you should take if flood warnings are broadcast.

- Make sure your battery radio is in working order and keep it tuned to a local station for instructions that will affect you. If the station should go off the air due to a power failure, tune to another station in the area.
- Make sure to have on hand emergency supplies of food, water, medical needs, and equipment – as well as extra batteries for all battery-operated equipment such as flashlights, radios, etc.

- Move furniture, electrical appliances, and other belongings to the upper floors of your house.
- Remove weed killers, insecticides, and all other poisonous materials of that nature to prevent polluting the water.
- If you have a toilet in your basement, remove the bowl and plug the toilet connection as well as the basement sewer drains. A bag of linseed or a wooden plug is ideal.
- Disconnect eavestroughing if it is connected to the house sewer system.
- Some homes may be protected by using sandbags or polyethylene barriers, but special methods must be used for each.

Don't attempt this type of protection without specific instructions from your local emergency officials.

If You're Forced Out

Should the flood waters rise to the point at which you are forced from you home, make sure you take essentials with you. These should include:
- Battery-powered radio and spare batteries.
- Flashlight with spare batteries.
- Warm clothing, waterproof outer garments and footwear, and blankets.
- Essential medicines, infant care items, personal toiletries, and as many emergency supplies as you have and can carry.
- Means of identification for each member of the family.
- Personal and family documents.

REMEMBER: if you are using your car, drive with extreme care.

After the Flood

Homes that are damaged by flooding need prompt clean-up action, but before entering a flood-damaged building, be sure it is not going to collapse. Rising flood waters can dislodge a building from its foundations, weaken walls, etc.

Do not turn on lights or appliances until an electrician has checked the electrical system for short circuits.

Wear rubber-soled boots and rubber gloves.

Stand on a dry board to turn off the main switch. Use a piece of rubber, plastic, or a dry stick to manipulate the metal handle of the switch box – do not touch the handle with your bare hand. Water in conduits or connection boxes, and dampness or exposed wires, can cause short circuits and fires. If any of these conditions exist and if you replace fuses, you could be electrocuted, especially if you are standing on a wet surface.

If a sump pump is available – and is needed – remove all fuses, except the main fuse and the one controlling the sump pump. Carefully turn on the main switch to find out if the pump operates. If not, call an electrician.

Flooding may have swollen doors tight. If an entrance must be forced because of swollen doors, accumulated mud, or bulged floors, use a window or other opening to get into the room. Take the pins out of the door hinges, make sure the door is unlocked, then go back outside and carefully push the door inward to avoid further damage.

Loose, wet ceiling plaster is heavy and dangerous. Knock down hanging plaster before moving around the building and watch for loose plaster as the building dries out.

Drying and Cleaning

Open doors and windows to permit air and heat to dry the house. To open swollen windows, remove the small strip that holds the lower sash. To accomplish this, use a chisel carefully so that you avoid marring the woodwork. Force the sash up slightly and remove it from the frame by pushing it from the outside into the hands of a helper inside the house. Be careful not to break the glass.

Examine the foundations and basement walls for signs of undermining. If settling and cracking has occurred, it may be necessary to dig down to the footings and reinforce or replace settled sections. Undermined footings should be reinforced with masonry or concrete, never with earth or gravel. Tilted or settled piers may need replacing. If the building is out of plumb, or the floors have settled or bulged, make sure that the foundation is sound and that there is no termite damage in sills, girders, and joists before beginning renovation. If the building must be moved, call in expert help.

Drain and clean the basement as soon as the building is safe. Pump or bail the water from the cellar and shovel out the mud while it is moist so that the basement floor can dry. Remove mud from the furnace, flues, and smoke-exhaust pipe.

Don't be in a rush to move back into the house. The house must be clean and dry before it is habitable.

Drain pools of water that may have accumulated in the premises. Remove and burn, or bury, any driftwood and rubbish, as well as decaying vegetation such as houseplants.

If the house or porches rest on open foundations, be sure the structure will not collapse before removing debris from underneath the building.

Walks and fences damaged by floodwaters are also a hazard until replaced or repaired.

Checking Heating Systems

If you have a *hot-air heating plant*, examine the inside of the heater. Wash sediment from the flues with a hose or a swab on a long stick. Generally, flues can be reached through the clean-out doors above the fire door. If the heater is jacketed, clean out all the mud between the stove and the outside casing, removing the casing if necessary.

If flues or passages are choked with mud, the boiler may burst when a fire is started. Take the smoke pipe out of the chimney and reach through the thimble to remove mud from the lower part of the chimney flue so that there will be a draft for the fire. An inadequate draft may fill the house with smoke or, worse, with deadly carbon monoxide gas.

If you have an *oil-burning system*, have the storage tank examined by an experienced inspector to make sure that seams have not opened, permitting dirt or water to enter. The burner should be dismantled and all parts cleaned in kerosene and wiped dry. Gear-housings should be removed and the gears thoroughly cleaned with kerosene. Any remaining grit will cause undue wear.

CAUTION
Burn kerosene-soaked rags out of doors. Do not wash them in an automatic washer; this may cause an explosion.

Small *electric motors* may be dried in an oven at not more than 65°C (150°F). If you are accustomed to working with electric motors, test them after six or eight hours of drying. If there is still evidence of grounding or short-circuiting, return the motor to the oven for another two to four hours before testing again.

CAUTION
If you are not accustomed to working with electric motors, do not risk electric shock by testing them yourself. Have the motors tested by a technician.

If your chimney was subjected to wind or water action, it should be inspected promptly. Defective chimneys can cause fires as well as carbon monoxide poisoning. Disintegrated mortar in the joints between bricks should be replaced with masonry cement. If the chimney has settled badly or broken where it passes though floors or roof, it may need rebuilding. If the chimney has settled or tilted, examine the footing to see if it has been undermined.

Safe Water Supply

Sanitary sewage disposal and a safe water supply are primary requirements for family health. If the water comes from a well, cistern, or a spring, ask your health department to check the water for safety – and have them tell you how to keep the source safe.

If water from a surface source must be used, take the supply from a point upstream from any inhabited area, dipping from well below the surface. Avoid sources with odours, dark colours, or floating material.

In an emergency, limited amounts of water may be obtained by draining a hot-water tank or by melting ice cubes.

There are two general methods for disinfecting small quantities of water – boiling and chemical treatment. Boiling is the best way to make water bacterially safe. Certain chemicals, if applied with care, will free most water of harmful or pathogenic organisms.

The effectiveness of the disinfectant method is reduced for water that is turbid or discoloured. First, filter such water through clean cloths or allow it to settle. Draw off the clear water to be disinfected and store it in clean, tightly covered, non-corrodible containers.

A ten-minute boiling will kill any disease-causing bacteria present. The flat taste of boiled water can be improved by allowing it to stand for a few hours, or by adding a small pinch of salt for each litre, or quart, of water boiled.

When boiling is not practical, a common practice is to add chlorine or iodine to the water. A chlorine solution may be prepared from one of three products:

- Consumer household bleach. Follow the instructions on the label; or find the percentage of chlorine in the solution as listed on the label and prepare the water following the proportions shown on this chart:

Available chlorine	Drops per litre (or quart) of clear water
1%	10
4-6%	2
7-10%	1

- If strength is unknown, add 10 drops per litre, or quart, to purify.
- Double the amount for turbid or coloured water.

Next mix the treated water thoroughly and allow it to stand for 30 minutes. If the water *does not* have a *slight* chlorine odour, repeat the dosage and allow it to stand for an additional 15 minutes.

The treated water may be made more palatable by allowing it to stand for several hours, or by pouring it back and forth a number of times between two clean containers.

- Granular calcium hypochlorite. Use 1 heaping teaspoon (1/4 ounce; 10 mL) with every 8 litres, or 2 gallons, of water. This makes a chlorine solution that can then be used to disinfect water.

  Add 1 part of the solution to each 100 parts of water, or roughly 0.5 litres to each 55 litres (or 1 pint to each 12.5 gallons).

- Chlorine tablets. These are available in commercially prepared form and may be obtained from drugstores and sporting goods stores. If there are no instructions on the package, use one tablet for each litre, or quart, of water.

Water can also be purified by either tincture of iodine or iodine tablets. Use five drops of 2% tincture of iodine to each litre, or quart, of clear water. For turbid water, use 10 drops and allow the solution to stand for at least 30 minutes.

Use commercially prepared iodine tablets according to the directions on the package, or add one tablet for each litre, or quart, of water.

All water used for drinking purposes, cooking, or brushing the teeth should be properly disinfected.

It is important to test plumbing and basement drains by pouring in a bucket of water. If the water does not run out, remove the clean-out plug from the trap and rake out the mud with a wire. Toilet and drain traps can be cleaned with water and a swab, or by rodding with a plumber's "snake" or a wire.

It may be necessary to disassemble and clean check-valves and other backflow preventers. In wind-damaged houses, all exposed pipes should be checked for intact connections before water is turned on.

Basement odours, although unpleasant, are usually harmless. If ventilation does not remove them, sprinkle bleaching powder (chloride of lime) on the floor. Allow it to remain until the floor dries, then sweep it up. This powder is a good disinfectant.

CAUTION

Bleaching powder is caustic and poisonous. Before sprinkling it on the basement floor, read the label on the container. Follow instructions and heed precautions. Keep bleaching powder out of the reach of children and away from eyes and mouth. Open doors and windows to provide ventilation while sprinkling the floor. Store the powder in a closed container away from moisture. Dispose of empty containers in a tightly covered refuse can.

Dry lump-charcoal kept in open containers may absorb odours from the air in enclosed spaces.

CAUTION

Charcoal is highly combustible when moist or wet, so guard against spontaneous combustion and fire. Expose only in tin cans or other containers made of hard metal. Keep well away from flammable liquids and gases, cloth, coal or firewood, or other readily combustible materials. Store charcoal in a well-ventilated place where it will remain dry and clean.

Mechanical Equipment

A competent technician should examine pump motors, refrigerators, freezers, ranges, washing machines, vacuum cleaners, food mixers, and other mechanical household equipment that has been exposed to water.

These appliances may be ruined if they are not cleaned and completely dry and free-running before the current is turned on.

Power washing-machines should be thoroughly cleaned before use. Open the gear housings and clean the shafts and gears with kerosene. Wipe all parts with a clean cloth, but be careful not to force any dirt into the bearings – even unseen grit can cause wear of moving parts. Wipe metal surfaces with a rag that has been dipped in kerosene to remove rust and dirt stains. Coat these surfaces thinly with petrolatum or machine oil to prevent further rusting. Before using the washer, oil the bearings. Then, with a soft cloth, dry all surfaces that were exposed to hands or clothing.

The cooling systems and motors of modern refrigerators are hermetically sealed. Their construction should rule out damage by immersion in water. In older refrigerators, however, the cooling unit is accessible and should be cleaned and examined.

For safety, technicians should inspect household machines and make necessary repairs, especially of motors and power-driven appliances.

Floors, Woodwork, Doors, and Roofs

After wet mud has been removed, floors may be badly buck-led. Do not attempt repairs until they are fully dry. Start the heating plant as soon as it will operate, but don't use so much heat that the house becomes steamy.

Dry the woodwork as fast as you can without aggravating shrinkage or deformation. Open windows and doors wide for good ventilation, but maintain a temperature of at least 10° to 15°C (50° to 60°F).

When the house is dry, some of the buckled flooring may be drawn back into place with nails. Some humps may be removed by planing or sanding. Heavily planed floors may never look good uncovered, but a smooth, old floor can serve as a base for new flooring. If smooth, an old floor may be covered with a resilient, smooth-surface floor covering. If the damage is too severe, new flooring may be necessary. If only the surface finish is damaged, the floor may be refinished.

Before the house has dried out, scrub woodwork with a stiff brush, plenty of water, and a detergent to remove mud and silt from corners and cracks. Drain accumulated water from partitions and exterior walls as quickly as possible so that insulation and structural members can dry.

Remove baseboards and drill holes between the studs a few inches above the floor. After the insulation and frames have dried, replace the baseboards.

For a final, thorough washing of floors, use the cleaning product you prefer – non-sudsing if possible. Don't do necessary refinishing until moisture has dried from the framing, from between walls and floors, and from the back of the trim – even though this may take months!

If any of the wood has become mildewed, use heat and ventilation to dry it. Badly infected wood may need to be replaced, preferably with wood that has been treated against mildew or that is naturally decay resistant.

Mildewed floors, woodwork, and other wooden areas may be scrubbed with a mild alkali, such as washing soda or trisodium phosphate. Use 4 to 5 tablespoons (2 to 3 ounces, or 50 to 90 mL) for every 4 litres (or 1 gallon) of water. Rinse well with clear water and allow the wood to dry thoroughly. Then apply a mildew-resistant paint.

CAUTION

Mildew-resistant paint contains fungicide and should not be used on playpens, cribs, or toys.

If mould has grown into the wood under paint or varnish, scrub it with an abrasive cleaner, then wash with a solution containing 4 to 6 tablespoons (2 to 3 ounces, or 50 to 90 mL) of trisodium phosphate and 1 cup (250 mL) of household chlorine bleach to 4 litres (1 gallon) of water. Rinse the wood well with clear water. Dry thoroughly and apply a wood preservative before repainting.

Locks, especially if made of iron, should be taken apart, wiped with kerosene, and oiled. If you cannot remove them, squirt a little machine oil through the bolt opening or the keyhole and work the knobs to distribute the oil. Otherwise, springs and metal casing will soon rust and need replacing. Do not use so much oil that it will drip onto the woodwork and make later painting difficult.

Hinges can usually be put back in order by cleaning and oiling.

Damaged roof covering can be repaired temporarily with material immediately at hand.

Plastered Walls and Wallpaper

Allow plaster to dry thoroughly before washing it. When it is dry, brush off any loose surface dirt, then wash painted walls with water and mild soap or any commercial cleaner (preferably non-sudsing).

Use two sponges and two buckets, one for the cleaning solution, the other for clear rinsing-water. Start washing the wall at the bottom and work up so that water will not run down and streak a soiled area. Water running down over a clean area can be wiped off without damage. Water running down over a soiled area will help set the stains.

Wash an area that you can reach easily without changing position; and rinse it immediately. Then wash the next area, overlapping the first. Proceed until the wall is finished. Badly stained walls will need redecorating. Ceilings should be done last.

After walls have been cleaned, and before wallpaper is replaced, paint or thoroughly spray the walls with a quaternary disinfectant, which you can find at dairy-supply outlets (if you have access to one) or a janitor-supply outlet. Add 1 ounce (2 tablespoons) of disinfectant to 8 litres (2 gallons) of water. This prevents mildew and may be applied both on painted walls and on washable wallpapers.

Often wallpaper is so discoloured and brittle from soaking that it must be removed and the walls repapered. If the wallpaper remained dry, but was loosened by dampness, it may be possible to repaste loosened edges or sections.

Clean the wallpaper with a commercial putty-like cleaner. Some wallpapers are washable, but if you are not sure whether the paper you are working on is, test a small inconspicuous spot using mild soap or synthetic detergent. If it is washable, proceed as you would for washing a painted wall. Squeeze as much water as possible out of the cleaning and rinsing sponges and *work quickly* so that the paper does not become soaked.

Grease spots may be removed from wallpaper with a paste of dry-cleaning fluid and cornstarch or talcum powder. Allow the paste to dry and then brush it off. Repeat if necessary.

CAUTION

Fumes from all dry-cleaning solvents are toxic and some are flammable. Use only with adequate ventilation, and read the precautions on the label.

Salvaging Furniture

Move wooden furniture outdoors and take out as many drawers, slides, or other working parts as possible.

Do not force stuck drawers with a screwdriver or chisel from the front. Remove the back – you may have to cut it out – and push out the drawers. Clean away all mud and dirt, using a stream of water from a hose if necessary. Then take the furniture back indoors and store it where it can dry slowly. Do not leave furniture in the sun as it will warp and twist out of shape.

Furniture made of solid wood may be salvaged by regluing. This may be difficult to do at home because many pieces require clamps. You might be better off taking it to a cabinetmaker.

Repairing veneered furniture is so difficult, and requires so many different types of tools, that it is not practical to try at home. A cabinetmaker is the answer, though you should check with the store where you purchased the furniture to determine whether the factory will make such repairs.

Furniture that has not been submerged may develop white spots or a whitish film or cloudiness due to the dampness. If the whole surface is affected, try rubbing it with a cloth wrung out in turpentine or camphorated oil. Wipe dry at once and polish with wax or furniture polish.

If the colour is not restored in this fashion, dip 3/0 steel wool in oil (boiled linseed, olive, mineral, or lemon) and rub lightly with the grain of the wood. Wipe with a soft cloth and rewax.

For deep spots, use a drop or two of ammonia on a damp cloth. Rub at once with a dry cloth, then polish.

Cigarette ashes rubbed in with your fingertips are often effective in removing white spots. If all efforts to remove white blemishes fail, refinishing may be the only solution.

Brush outer coverings of upholstered articles, mattresses, rugs, and carpets to remove loose mould. Do this outdoors to prevent scattering mildew spores in the house. Run a vacuum-cleaner attachment over the surface. Dry the article with an electric heater or fan, or any convenient method. Then sun and air the article to prevent mould growth.

If mildew remains, sponge upholstery or mattresses lightly with thick suds of soap or synthetic detergent, then wipe with a clean, damp cloth. Use little water on the fabric to avoid soaking the padding.

Another way of cleaning upholstered furniture is to wipe it with a cloth wrung out of diluted alcohol (equal parts of denatured or rubbing alcohol and water). Then dry the article thoroughly.

With a low-pressure spray containing a fungicide, moisten mildewed surfaces thoroughly. Aerosol spraying is not effective in controlling fungi.

CAUTION

Do not inhale mist from a spray or use it near flame. Follow all precautions on the packaged product.

In closed areas, vapours of paradichlorobenzene or paraformaldehyde will stop mould growth. If moulds have grown into the article, it should be dried and fumigated by a dry-cleaning or storage company. Fumigation will kill existing mould but will not protect the article in future.

Badly damaged upholstered furniture that has been submerged may need restuffing. Springs may need to be cleaned and oiled and the frame may need cleaning.

Metals

Clean metal at once, especially iron. Wipe rust from iron with a kerosene-soaked cloth. Coat iron hardware lightly with petrolatum or machine oil to prevent further rusting. Use stove polish on stoves and similar ironwork.

Wash cooking utensils thoroughly with soapy water to remove kerosene, then rub with unsalted cooking fat and heat very slowly to permit the fat to soak the pores of the metal for rust resistance.

Stainless steel, nickel-copper alloy, or metals plated with nickel or chromium need only thorough washing and polishing with a fine-powdered cleanser. If the plating is broken, thus exposing the base metal to rust, wipe with kerosene, wash and dry the surface, and then wax for rust resistance.

Wash aluminum thoroughly and scour unpolished surfaces with soap-filled metal scouring pads. Polished or plated surfaces of aluminum should be wiped with silver polish or fine cleaning powder.

To brighten darkened insides of aluminum pans, fill with water, add 50 mL (2 ounces, or 1/4 cup) of vinegar or 15 mL (1/2 ounce, or 1 tablespoon) of cream of tartar for each litre (or quart) of water; boil for 10 to 15 minutes. Then scour with a soap-filled pad. If utensils have been submerged in flood water and are darkened both inside and out, prepare one of the above-mentioned acid solutions in a large container and immerse them; then proceed with the treatment described.

Copper and brass can be polished with a special polish sold for that purpose, or with salt sprinkled on a piece of lemon or on a cloth saturated with vinegar. Wash utensils thoroughly after treatment.

Earthquakes: Be Prepared

FORTUNATELY, EARTHQUAKES do not often occur in urban areas in Canada. But this does not mean they never happen. Depending on what part of the country you live in, there is a chance that your area could be hit by an earthquake.

You can see from the map below which areas of this country are most vulnerable. And if you live in a risk area you will want to know two things: what to expect and what to do if an earthquake occurs.

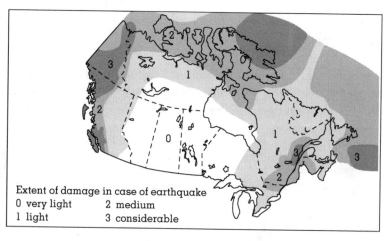

Extent of damage in case of earthquake
0 very light   2 medium
1 light   3 considerable

The map shows those areas of Canada susceptible to earthquakes.

What Could Happen

An earthquake is often announced by a loud noise not unlike that of an oncoming train. Initial earth movements and swaying of structures caused by an earthquake can be followed some time later (often hours; sometimes days) by aftershocks, usually of decreasing severity.

The actual movement of the ground during an earthquake is not the thing to fear most. History has shown us that this awesome movement underfoot is seldom the direct cause of death or injury. Most casualties result from falling objects and debris. The earthshocks shake, damage, or demolish buildings and other structures. Earthquakes have also been known to trigger earthslides and to generate huge ocean waves – called *tsunamis*, or seismic sea waves – either of which can cause horrendous damage.

Buildings don't automatically collapse during earthquakes. Some, such as timber frame houses, may withstand the earth shock very well. But it is true that chimneys, parapets, ceiling plaster, and light fixtures may fall. There can be flying glass from broken windows. Fires may be caused by broken chimneys and gas lines. Broken water mains can aggravate the dangers. Fallen power lines are not only an electrical hazard, especially if there is water in the streets. Following the earth's upheaval, downed electrical lines can leave communities without power for days.

How To Be Prepared

There are many things you can do to reduce the dangers of earthquakes.

- Check your home for earthquake hazards. Bolt down or provide other strong support for water heaters and gas appliances. Fire damage can result from broken gas lines and appliance connections. Use flexible connections wherever possible. Place large or heavy objects on lower shelves of cupboards, bookcases, etc.
- In new construction and alterations, follow building codes to minimize earthquake hazards. Sites for construction should

be selected and engineered to reduce the hazard of damage from an earthquake.

- Plan ahead. Hold occasional earthquake drills to ensure that your family knows what to do. This could avoid injury and panic in the event of an earthquake.
- Teach responsible family members how to turn off electricity at the main switch, and gas and water at the main valves.
- Ensure that responsible members of your family know first-aid techniques. Hospitals and clinics could be overloaded after a severe earthquake.
- Always have a battery-powered radio handy, as well as a flashlight. And have spare batteries for both.
- Always keep on hand an emergency survival kit containing food (see page 100 for suggested food supplies; you might need enough for four or five days), sleeping bags, medication, first-aid supplies, and bottled water. Rotate food and water to ensure freshness. If you must leave home during or after an earthquake, take along with you this kit, as well as your portable radio and your flashlight.

If an Earthquake Occurs

Try to *stay calm*. Do *not* panic! If you are indoors, stay there. Don't run outside the moment the earth begins to shake. You could be hit by falling glass and debris.

If you are in a house, a store, or a high-rise building, take cover under a heavy piece of furniture – a desk, table, bed, or overturned piece of upholstered furniture such as a sofa; or stand in an inside doorway, away from windows. A door frame and inner core of a building are its strongest points and least likely to collapse.

Don't dash for an exit. Remember, stairways may have collapsed or could be jammed with people. And if the power fails, elevators stop running, even if they're between floors high up in a building.

If you are outside, stay there. Move away from buildings to avoid crumbling walls and falling debris. Stay away from power lines and dangling electric wires.

If you are driving your car, stop immediately and stay in the vehicle. If possible, do not stop on a bridge or an overpass, or where buildings could tumble down on you. Your car can provide protection from falling debris.

After an Earthquake

If you are not injured and don't need assistance, you can be useful.

- Listen to your battery-operated or car radio for instructions. Follow them.
- Check for fires. In case of fire, notify the fire department. Try to control small fires until help comes.
- Give first aid to injured persons; get help if necessary. Help others who may be trapped by debris. Exercise caution – don't injure yourself.
- Do *not* enter or re-enter damaged buildings; walls may yet collapse after the original shaking has ceased.
- Check all utilities; look for broken water pipes, shorting electrical circuits, or leaking heating fuel. Do *not* use a match or open flame to find your way. If you find or even suspect damage, shut off utilities at main valves or meter boxes. Turn off heating appliances and check for damage.
- Don't use the telephone except in a real emergency. Leave the lines open for official use.
- If water is off, use emergency water from water heaters, toilet tanks, melted ice cubes, and canned vegetables.
- Check that sewage lines are intact before permitting continued flushing of toilets.
- If power is off, plan to use foods from your freezer before they spoil. Outdoor charcoal broilers can be used for emergency cooking.
- Check chimneys for cracks, especially in the attic and at the roof line. Unnoticed damage can lead to a fire.
- Don't go sightseeing. Drive your car only if vitally necessary, and then with caution. Keep the roads clear for rescue and emergency vehicles. Do not enter damaged areas unless you have been asked by officials to do so.

- Keep your emergency supplies, clothing, and food handy in case you are called on to evacuate the area. If it becomes necessary to evacuate homes, you will be advised.
- Wear shoes in all areas near debris and broken glass.
- Stay away from waterfront areas. Large earthquakes at sea are often followed by a *tsunami*, often incorrectly referred to as a "tidal wave."

CHAPTER 7

Nuclear Emergency

A GENERATION AGO, much of the planning about survival in the event of a nuclear emergency centred on what to do in the event of a war. Today, planning for a nuclear emergency is more concerned with how to cope in the event a nuclear power generating station has an accident.

We have been made sensitively aware in recent years of such accidents both close to home – Three Mile Island in the United States – and on the other side of the globe – Chernobyl in the Soviet Union. And while the nuclear stations being built today are designed to be safe, it is still important to be ready for an emergency.

A nuclear emergency could result from a release of radioactivity from a nuclear generating station into the environment. Such an occurrence would affect people living around that station and as far as 10 kilometres (about 6.25 miles) away. Some experts feel precautions should be taken in an area as far as 16 km (10 miles) from a nuclear power station and others feel the safety zone should be extended to double that distance.

Unlike a situation in which a nuclear bomb is set off, there will be no explosion or even the threat of an explosion should a problem develop at a nuclear power generating station. It is highly likely that there would be several hours' advance notice, even in the worst emergency, before any release of radioactivity from the station. That would provide most area residents with sufficient time to ensure their safety.

Various governmental bodies have planned to provide information to the populace should such an emergency occur. Radio and TV stations have been designated to carry news of such a disaster as well as action plans. But even if you are not tuned in, you will be alerted by police who will tour the affected neighbourhoods with sirens and loudspeakers. There will probably also be door-to-door visits by emergency personnel.

Nuclear generating stations in this country are built with a series of safeguards ensuring that radioactive materials are kept within the plant. These safeguards are maintained by careful plant operation, regular testing of equipment and components, and operators who are trained (and get repeated re-training) to respond to emergency conditions. In the event of an accident, special safety systems also provide extra methods of defence.

We are exposed to radiation daily. It is common in nature and has always existed. Radiation is found in plants and animals, in the air we breathe, and in the food we eat. Even our own bodies contain natural radiation in the form of radioactive carbon and potassium.

Radiation is measured in units called "rems" and "millirems," which are 1/1000th of a rem. A rem is a measure of radiation indicating potential effects on human cells. A millirem is the unit used to measure radiation dosage. For example, watching colour TV exposes us to one millirem in a year. Taking a cross-country flight exposes us to five millirems. A medical or dental x-ray picture exposes us to 100 millirems. The average exposure to living in highly industrialized areas of the country is about 300 millirems a year from both natural and man-made sources of radiation.

In the event of a nuclear accident, protective action would begin if the radiation exposure was expected to be more than 100 millirems – the same level one is exposed to with a single x-ray picture for medical purposes.

What You May Need To Do

Should there be an emergency at a nuclear generating station in your community, you may be required to stay indoors, keeping your doors and windows closed. Staying indoors is a most effective way of reducing exposure to low levels of radioactive materials that can be released from a nuclear generating station. Keeping the doors and windows closed would reduce the exposure to radiation by perhaps 40 per cent.

Be prepared for the following decisions to be made by the authorities:
• School and business activities will probably be suspended.
• Routine admissions to hospital may be suspended.
• Traffic into the area may be restricted.
• There may be an evacuation of the affected area.

If you are to remain in your home, you will probably be told to shower to remove low-level radioactive dust particles. This is essential if you were outdoors during the time of the emergency. Even though the radiation levels would be low, it is still wise to take the following precautions.
1. Remove your clothes and place them in a plastic bag that should then be sealed.
2. Take a shower and thoroughly rinse your body and hair.
3. Put on clean clothes that have been in a closet or drawer that has been closed. After the emergency is over, the clothes should be monitored for radioactivity. If there is any sign of radioactivity, the clothes will need cleaning.

You will be advised to avoid foods and liquids that have become contaminated by radioactive particles. This includes vegetables from your garden, locally produced milk, and any foods that were on display or were not packaged at the time of the accident. If you live on a farm, animals should be prevented from taking food or water that may have become contaminated.

You may be provided with potassium iodine pills to protect your thyroid gland from radioactive iodine. When a person breathes radioactive iodine in air, it enters the bloodstream and is absorbed and stored by the thyroid gland. An effective means of preventing the thyroid from absorbing the radioactive iodine is the potassium iodine pill. What happens is that the iodine from the pill fills the thyroid, causing it to temporarily stop accumulating radioactive iodine. The radioactive iodine is then flushed from the body naturally.

Potassium iodine pills can be ordered through your pharmacist and kept in a safe, childproof place against the day when they may be needed. They will also be available from emergency authorities when the need arises. But they should only be taken when advised by your doctor or by emergency authorities. They do not protect the body from other radioactive materials. That means that simply taking the pills does not provide complete protection. You must still take shelter and shower as protection against other radioactivity.

Protecting Loved Ones

Do not try to pick up children from school if an emergency is declared and you are asked to stay indoors or to evacuate the area.

The Board of Education in your community will have a plan to take care of all children in its care. Each school has its own procedures for responding to all types of emergencies, including nuclear emergency. If you have children in private school or a day-care centre, check with their officials now about what their plans are.

Should evacuation be necessary, children will be reunited with families as soon as possible. And information about their whereabouts will be broadcast and will be available as well from emergency authorities.

Other family members who are not at home but are within the area affected by the emergency may be evacuated to centres that are set up for the purpose. Family members will be reunited as quickly as possible. You can be reassured that hospitals, homes for the aged, nursing homes, and other live-in institutions have their own emergency plans. If you have family members in any of these institutions, you should check now about what their plans are.

If an emergency occurs and you find that you need assistance because you are elderly, or ill, or physically disabled, wrap a white cloth (towel, shirt, sheet, etc.) around an outside doorknob or hang it from a window that is visible from the street. Police patrolling the area will see this distress signal and ensure that assistance is provided.

Taking Shelter Indoors

If you are advised to take shelter indoors following a nuclear emergency:

- *Do not* try to pick up children at school – they will be looked after.
- *Do not* use the telephone – leave the lines free for official use.
- Stay calm.
- Get people and pets indoors.
- Close doors and windows.
- Turn on radio or TV to a station designated to carry emergency information.
- Minimize air entering the house from outside. During warm weather, turn off the air conditioning; during the heating season, turn the thermostat down to 15°C (60°F).
- Turn off stoves and put out fires in fireplaces. Allow smoke to escape up the chimney, then close dampers.
- If you were outside when the emergency occurred, remove your clothes and seal them in a plastic bag. Get into the shower and wash body and hair. When you put on clean clothes, take them from a closet or drawer that was closed.
- Move to the centre of the house or into the basement.
- Stay indoors until advised otherwise.
- If you must go outside for any urgent reason, make the trip as brief as possible. Then shower immediately after you return and follow the same procedure about clothing that you did if you were outside when the emergency occurred.

If Evacuation Is Necessary

The authorities may notify residents of the endangered area to evacuate. Those instructions will be broadcast over radio and TV stations that are designated to carry emergency broadcasts. In addition, police cars will tour all communities affected and will announce through their loudspeaker systems that evacuation has been ordered.

Should this situation occur, remember, you must not try to pick up family members from schools, hospitals, nursing homes, or other institutions. They will be looked after carefully.

If your vehicle is in poor running condition, or nearly out of gas, *do not* take it out onto the road. Instead, stay indoors and signal for assistance with a white cloth, as discussed above.

Before you leave the house, turn off all appliances except the refrigerator and freezer. Do not turn off the gas service to your house unless specifically instructed to do so. And, as you would if you were taking shelter indoors, turn off the air conditioner in warm weather, or turn your thermostat down to 15°C or 60°F in cold weather. Then lock windows and doors.

If you have livestock, shelter them where possible and provide food and water for several days. Leave pets indoors and also leave enough food and water for them for two days. You will be allowed to come back and look after them as soon as possible.

If possible, leave in company with neighbours. Remember to offer assistance to anyone who needs it. Tune your car radio to an emergency station and listen for instructions.

Leave the area along designated routes. Head for your area's emergency reception centre where information will be made available as to the whereabouts of other members of your family.

All evacuated areas will be kept under tight security. Unauthorized persons will not be allowed into evacuated areas. Police may reroute traffic and restrict entry to certain areas in order to keep main traffic arteries free for evacuation. You will be advised when you can return home.

What To Take With You

Before leaving your house pack essential items. These include:
- Extra clothing
- Baby supplies and special food
- Toilet articles
- Blankets
- Eyeglasses and dentures
- Prescription drugs and important medicines
- Driver's licence and identification
- Chequebook, credit cards, and cash.

CHAPTER 8

The Bomb and After

GOVERNMENTS AND COMMUNITIES at all levels have plans for the survival of mankind in the event of a nuclear war. True, casualties will grow to horrendous numbers if there is even a limited nuclear war. But the survival of individuals could depend in great part on the preparation that each person makes.

Part of that preparation should include knowing what your municipality has as its war-emergency plan. Most municipalities in Canada have emergency plans to deal both with peacetime disasters and with nuclear-attack situations.

This would be true whether you plan to go to a designated shelter before an anticipated attack or to remain at home. You should know what arrangements are in place to instruct the public about staying in shelter and about coming out of shelter when it is considered safe. When the sirens or other warning devices sound and your local radio station confirms that an attack on this continent has been detected, will you recognize the "attack warning" signal? Will you know where to turn on your radio or television to listen for instructions? Will you know where to take shelter? Will you know how to take shelter? Thinking about the problems with which you could be faced should a nuclear attack be launched against North America is the first important step.

Blast, light, heat, and *radioactive fallout* are the primary problems. Fallout also is a very serious health hazard. Counter-measures for personal and family protection include the need for assessment of radiation, as well as advice and instructions. A workable survival plan will include all the preparations you can make in advance to meet these problems.

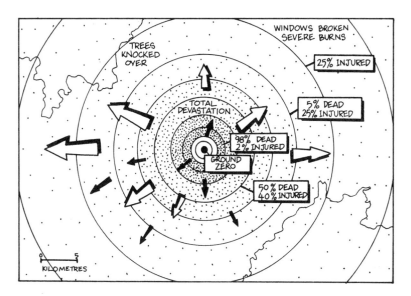

The area damaged in a nuclear-bomb explosion diminishes outward from "ground zero" – the point of the blast.

Nuclear Explosions

A five-megaton H-bomb – that is, a bomb with the explosive force of five million tons of dynamite – could substantially damage the largest Canadian city. And that's the kind of weapon we can expect in the event of a nuclear war.

The explosion releases vast amounts of energy in three forms: light and heat, blast, radiation. The effects depend on whether a weapon explodes high in the air or near the ground. An air burst usually produces more fire- and blast-damage than a ground burst. On the other hand, a ground burst results in a greater amount of radioactive fallout, and a huge crater.

A blaze of light, brighter than the sun, is produced by a nuclear explosion. It lasts about 15 seconds. Temporary or permanent blindness and eye injury can result from the glare if your eyes are not shielded.

The heat rays from the explosion travel at the speed of light: 186,000 miles (almost 300,000 kilometres) a second. It can start fires up to 22 miles (35 kilometres) away. Many household fires are triggered when the "heat pulse" comes through a window, igniting draperies, curtains, paper, clothing, rugs, and furniture. The heat flash can also set fire to the outside of wooden buildings. If a five-megaton bomb were exploded on a clear day, this is what happens to unprotected skin:

• At 15 miles (25 kilometres) it is badly burned.
• At 18 miles (30 kilometres) it blisters.
• At 23 miles (37 kilometres) the burns resemble a bad sunburn.

If the explosion takes place in the air, rather than on the ground, there is a greater chance of serious burns from the heat flash. Clothing gives protection. If there is a building or other form of "shield" between a person and the flash, it, too, will give protection against burns.

The "blast wave" travels more slowly than the heat flash. Several seconds may pass, after the light and the heat, before the blast wave reaches you – in much the same way as lightning and thunder – depending on the distance you are from the explosion, it would take about 35 seconds for the blast wave to reach you. If you are caught in the open at the time of a nuclear explosion, that half-minute or so can be used to find some protection from the blast wave.

You could be injured by being thrown about by the blast. Therefore, *keep low*. The greatest danger is from flying glass, bricks, and other debris. The blast from a five-megaton bomb could injure you if you are as far away as 15 miles or 25 kilometres.

Buildings and everything else within three miles (five kilometres) of the centre of the explosion would be completely destroyed. Buildings three to five miles (five to eight kilometres) from the blast would be damaged beyond repair. Major repairs would be required before buildings five to ten miles (eight to 15 kilometres) away could be occupied again. Light to moderate damage would be done to buildings 10 to 15 miles (15 to 25 kilometres) distant.

If the bomb were four times as large – a 20-megaton variety – the range at which the damage described could be done increases to five, eight, sixteen, and twenty-five miles (eight, thirteen, twenty-six, and forty kilometres), respectively.

These are all approximate distances because the strength of buildings is not uniform. Reinforced concrete buildings are obviously more blast-resistant than wood-frame structures. Windows are, of course, extremely vulnerable. They could be blown in as far as 25 miles (40 kilometres) from the explosion.

The explosion causes two kinds of radiation: immediate and residual. *Immediate radiation*, as its name implies, is emitted at the time of the explosion. It is dangerous only within two to three miles (three to five kilometres). You might be able to survive the blast if you were near the explosion without adequate protection, but you would be seriously affected by the immediate radiation. *Residual radiation* is given off by the radioactive particles left by "fallout" after the explosion. The danger from fallout can be great and widespread.

Radioactive Fallout

Fallout danger is greater if the bomb is exploded on, or near, the ground. The force of the explosion itself could make a crater up to one mile (1.5 kilometres) wide and 100 feet (30 metres) deep. Millions of tons of pulverized earth, stone, buildings, and other materials will be drawn up into the fireball and become radioactive.

This radioactive material is then carried by the winds until it settles back to earth. Under some circumstances you might see the fallout, under others you will not. The radioactivity it gives off *cannot* be seen. You can't feel it. You can't smell it.

Fallout doesn't come out of the sky like a gas and seep into everything. It has been described as "a fine to coarse sand" carried by the winds. Because wind direction varies at different heights, it is not possible to judge from the ground where the fallout will settle. It can settle in irregular patterns, hundreds of miles from the explosion.

An area of 7,000 square miles (12,000 square kilometres) could be seriously affected by a five-megaton bomb. That's more than three times the size of Prince Edward Island. There would be grave danger to life in that area.

Four things determine the amount of radiation that can reach your body from fallout:
• The *time that has passed* since the explosion.
• The *amount of time you are exposed* to fallout.
• The *distance* you are from the fallout.
• The *shielding* between you and the fallout.

The radioactivity in fallout weakens rapidly in the first hours after an explosion. After seven hours, this "decay" results in a loss of about 90 per cent of the strength it had one hour after the explosion. After two days it has lost 99 per cent. In two weeks, 99.9 per cent of its strength is gone. However, if the radiation at the beginning was high enough, the remaining 0.1 per cent can still be extremely dangerous.

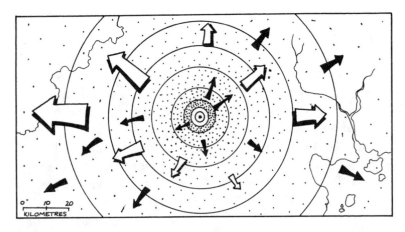

Radioactive material will carry in all directions – but fallout will travel farther in some directions due to prevailing winds.

CAUTION

Stay in your shelter until radiation has been measured by the authorities, and until you have been told over the radio or television that it is safe to come out.

The farther you are from the fallout, the weaker will be the radiation reaching your body. The most effective protection you can have is heavy material between yourself and the fallout. The heavier the material, the better the protection.

Ninety-nine per cent of radiation can be stopped by the following thicknesses of common materials:
• Three inches (eight centimetres) of lead.
• Five inches (13 centimetres) of steel.
• Sixteen inches (40 centimetres) of solid brick.
• Sixteen inches (40 centimetres) of hollow concrete blocks filled with mortar or sand.
• Two feet (60 centimetres) of packed earth.
• Three feet (one metre) of loose earth.
• Three feet (one metre) of water.

A fallout shelter is the best way to protect your family and yourself against radiation. It keeps the radiation at a distance; it shields you from the radiation; and it keeps you under a protective wrap during the time that the radiation is most intense. If you provide yourself with a fallout shelter, you are unlikely to suffer serious effects from radioactive fallout.

Radioactive particles in contact with your skin for a few hours may produce burns. If swallowed in food or water, they could be harmful. An unprotected person could become ill after a few days. The illness develops slowly, though it is not infectious – that is, it cannot be spread from one person to another.

Except for temporary nausea shortly after exposure, evidence of serious effects of exposure may only appear after an interval ranging from a few days to three weeks. A combination of loss of hair, loss of appetite, increasing paleness, weakness, diarrhea, sore throat, bleeding gums, and easy bruising indicate that you require medical attention.

Remember, however, that nausea and vomiting may be caused by fright, worry, food poisoning, pregnancy, and other common conditions.

Recognize the Warning

All communities in this country, where there is a likely need, have been provided with sirens. In some areas there are warning systems consisting of horns, bells, or factory whistles. These devices are only meant as attention-getters. When you hear the warning signal, *take protective action* and *listen to the radio* for instructions.

Take a battery-powered radio with you; and take extra batteries! Broadcast advice and instruction may help save your life. If you don't have a portable radio, turn up the volume of your house radio so that you can hear it from your shelter. If you are in your car away from home and are able to take shelter nearby, turn up the volume and open all the vehicle's doors or windows. You will soon be told over the Canadian Emergency Broadcast System when and how to take emergency protective action.

If the warnings are for impending attack, regardless of where you are or what you are doing, you *must* take the best available cover against the blast, heat, and light effects of nuclear explosion. Emergency broadcast instructions will include the following advice:

- If you are at home go to the basement or strongest part of the building. If material is handy, improvise blast protection. (See pages 97-99.)
- Take your battery radio with you (with extra batteries), or turn up the house radio so that you can hear it while under cover.
- Stay away from windows.
- Lie down to protect yourself from flying glass and debris.
- Shield your eyes from the flash.

- If you are away from home, take protective cover immediately.
- If you are travelling, stop and take protective cover immediately. *If* you are only a few minutes away from a safe destination, proceed; then take protective cover immediately.
- Listen to your radio for further instructions.

If the warnings continue to sound after an attack, it could mean another attack, or it could mean that radioactive fallout is nearing your area. *You will be advised over the radio.* If the advice concerns fallout, you must immediately take cover to avoid its effects.

Radio broadcasts will identify areas that will be affected by the fallout and give instructions and advice. This might include:
- Location of explosions causing fallout locally.
- Location of parts of the country to be affected by fallout.
- Length of time before fallout is expected to reach specific area.
- Ways to increase fallout protection.
- Supplies to take to your fallout shelter.
- Advice on whether it is safe to stay where you are or go to some other area.
- Advice as to what areas are free of danger.
- Advice on conservation of food, water, and fuel.
- Advice on keeping warm should power be cut in cold weather.
- Requests for assistance.

CAUTION

Do not use the telephone. All telephone lines will be required for official use. Listen to your radio or television for information.

How To Take Shelter

Assuming that you have not built a bomb shelter in your home, you should know how to improvise. One of the simplest ways to improvise some anti-blast protection is to build a lean-to, made of bed springs or boards against a workbench or heavy table, preferably in the basement. Then pile mattresses on top of it and at the ends. If this material is readily available, it could be built in a matter of minutes after the attack warning is sounded and it could protect you from loose bricks, flying glass, falling debris, etc.

Another way of improvising a shelter is to use furniture, doors, dressers, or other such materials. Select a corner of your basement, if possible away from the windows, in which to build the shelter.

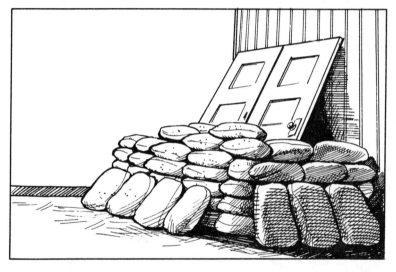

A simple, effective bomb shelter consists of doors leaned against a concrete wall reinforced with bags of earth or sand.

Remove the hinges from inside house doors so that the doors can be used as a shelter-roof over supports. These supports can be cabinets, chests of drawers, a workbench, or anything that can bear a heavy load. Use the doors as a roof surface to provide a base for the heavy material you are going to put on top of them. Bricks, concrete blocks, sand-filled drawers or boxes, books, or other dense items on this roof will help reduce radiation penetration. Around the sides and front of your shelter, build walls of dense materials to provide vertical shielding. A small cabinet or dirt-filled box may be used in a crawl-in entrance as a "door" that can be pulled closed behind you. Remember that the heavier or more dense the material around you, the greater the protection. Use earth, concrete, brick, books, or even bundles of newspapers to block basement windows. In winter, packed snow will serve as well.

On the floor above the basement, over the corner you selected for your shelter, pile any heavy objects you may have available – furniture, trunks filled with clothes, dirt-filled boxes, books, newspaper, or earth from outside. And outside the house, against the walls of the basement around your shelter area, heap earth, sand, bricks, concrete blocks, or even packed snow.

If your home has no basement or crawl space, build your emergency shelter in that part of the house (centre hall or clothes closet) farthest from the outside walls and the roof. Build it the same way as was described for the basement shelter. And on the floor *immediately above the shelter,* follow the same advice as for the floor above a basement shelter.

If you are in the open and there is a ditch or a culvert within quick easy reach, lie face down in it and cover your face with your arms. Make sure this shelter is not too close to buildings that could collapse into it. After the blast and the heat of the explosion, you will have to find other protection against fallout that will come later.

Emergency Supplies

It may be advisable to stay in your shelter for *14 days*. That means preparing supplies to last you for two weeks. These supplies should include food, water, battery-powered radio, battery-powered lights, first-aid kit, necessary medical supplies, extra batteries for your radio and lights, as well as heavy clothing (depending on the season) and extra changes of clothing, particularly stockings and underclothing.

Remember, if you have children with you, you should take things to occupy their time in the shelter – books, toys, games, etc.

Civil defence authorities have prepared the following suggested list of things to take with you for the two-week stay in shelter.

Equipment

Beds (bunks or folding)	Toilet
Bedding	Polyethylene bags for toilet
Table (folding or other)	Paper towels
Stools (folding)	Garbage can (two, if no waste
Cups and plates (disposable)	water runoff is possible)
Knives, forks, spoons	Garbage bags
Can opener	Shovel
Cooking utensils	Broom
Kerosene cooker*	Battery radio, spare batteries
Kerosene (for 14 days)	Electric lamp, spare bulbs
Candles and holder	Flashlight (or battery lamp),
Safety matches	spare batteries and bulbs
Hand basin	Clock
Calendar	Fire extinguisher
Pocket knife	Hand tools, axe
String	Light rope

CAUTION

----

*Do not use a pressurized stove in the confines of your shelter.

Food

The following amounts are for *one* adult for *14 days*. As you stock these items in your shelter, mark the purchase date on them. Food stored for emergency purposes should be used and replaced at least once a year.

Milk: 14 cans (160 mL; 6 oz) or 6 cans (385 mL; 15 oz) evaporated milk or (500 g; 1 lb) dried skim milk

Vegetables: 6 cans (398 or 540 mL; 15 or 20 oz) beans, peas, tomatoes, corn

Fruit: 6 cans (398 or 540 mL; 15 or 20 oz) peaches,
                  pears, apple sauce
Juices: 6 cans (540 mL; 20 oz) apple, grapefruit, lemon,
                  orange, tomato
Cereals: 14 individual packages (sealed in wax bags inside
                  or outside)
Biscuits: 2 packages of crackers (450 g; 1 lb) each
                  2 packages cookies or graham wafers
Main Dish: 2 cans (340 g; 12 oz) corned beef, luncheon meats
                  2 cans beef and gravy
                  2 cans baked beans (398 or 540 mL; 15 or 20 oz)
                  2 jars cheese
                  2 cans fish (227 mL; 8 oz)
Soup: 2 cans (284 mL; 10 oz) bean, pea, tomato, vegetable
Other: 1 large jar or can honey, syrup, jam, or marmalade
                  1 package (450 g; 1 lb) hard candy
                  1 jar or can peanut butter
                  1 package tea bags or instant tea
                  1 jar instant coffee
                  1 jar sugar
                  Salt and pepper
                  Instant chocolate powder
                  Chewing gum

Special Requirements for Children

- For *each infant* include 14 cans (385 mL; 15 oz) evaporated milk and infant food for 14 days.
- For *each child up to three years*, include 8 extra cans of milk.
- Decrease amounts of other foods according to appetite.
- Food for older children can be the same as for adults; adjust amounts according to appetite.

Water

Requirements: 7-14 gallons (32-64 litres) for each adult; more for younger children (some water may be replaced by canned beverages).

Containers: Store water in well-cleaned, covered containers such as thermos jugs, new fuel cans, large bottles, or plastic containers.

Change: Change stored water at least once a month.

Toiletries

Soap, toothpaste
Toothbrushes
Detergent
Nail brush
Razor, blades, and soap

Women's basic cosmetics
Tissues (face and toilet)
Face cloths
Towels
Comb and brush

Clothing and Personal Items

Coveralls, rubber boots, rubber gloves for adults – to be used in venturing outside even after instructions have been given that this is safe for short periods.

Bedding (blankets preferable)
Warm sweaters and socks
Change of underclothing, socks
Personal hygiene items for women
Legal papers

Baby clothes
Baby feeding equipment
Disposable diapers (for 2 weeks)
Plastic Sheeting

Medical Supplies

A simple first-aid box kept in your shelter, or in your evacuation kit, should contain:

1 bottle mild antiseptic solution for cleaning cuts

1 package 2" (5 cm) gauze bandage

2 triangular bandages for use as slings

1 package 4" x 4" (10 cm x 10 cm) sterile pads to cover cuts, wounds, and burns

1 package assorted adhesive dressings for minor cuts

1 roll adhesive tape

1 small bottle toothache drops

1 small bottle ASA (Aspirin) tablets or acetaminophen (Tylenol) tablets

Petroleum jelly

Assorted safety pins
Oral thermometer (and rectal, if required)
Small, blunt-ended scissors
Medicine glass
Tweezers
Small package baking soda and small package table salt to make an anti-shock drinking solution by adding 1 tsp salt and 1/2 tsp baking soda to 1 quart (1 litre) water
First-aid manual

CAUTION

Make sure you take with you any medication anyone in the family may need. If anyone requires special medication such as insulin, be sure to maintain at least a three-month supply.

Recreational

Books	Chess, checkers, other games
Paper	Crosswords, other puzzles
Pencils and sharpener	Knitting, sewing, etc.
Playing cards	Hobby materials, plasticine

Fires

Misinformation about fire danger from nuclear explosions is widespread and common. For example, some people believe that the fireball would completely incinerate a city. This is not true. The heat from the fireball lasts about 15 seconds. It will create fires that are no different from any other kind of fires. They can be put out with water and extinguishers, and if each survivor were able to put out a small fire quickly, mass fires probably would not develop,

As we said earlier, the heat flash entering through windows could set fire to draperies, rugs, furniture, clothing, or piles of paper. Other fires could break out in the attic, in backyard trash, on wooden shingles, and on the outsides of houses built of wood, especially if they are unpainted or weathered.

Knowing how to prevent and fight fires at home and at work reduces the number of peacetime fires. The same knowledge will also reduce the number of fires caused by a nuclear explosion.

But how can you fight fires in the presence of fallout? Between five and 15 miles (eight and 25 kilometres) from the centre of the explosion, there will be many survivors. Fallout will not start coming down for about 30 minutes. During this half-hour, survivors should inspect their homes and put out all small fires they can. They must not rely on the fire department to extinguish these fires.

You should have in your home and place of work fire extinguishers (see Chapter One). In an emergency, create a water supply for fire-fighting by using pails, bathtubs, washtubs, etc. Don't rely on being able to use the established water supply system. Even people living in areas not attacked may find their fire departments will have to fight major fires elsewhere.

To prepare for an emergency, here are some things you should know:
- Prevent accumulations of trash and rubbish in and around the house. This includes dry leaves and grass, lumber, boxes, cartons, unused furniture, bales of newspapers, etc. Keep waste and garbage in covered containers.
- The shaking and twisting of buildings due to blast waves in wartime, or earthquakes and explosions at other times, may break utility inlets at the point they enter the structure. This may allow gas or fuel oil to flow into basements, creating a severe hazard. Therefore *do not* smoke, strike a match, or use a lighter to light your way into a darkened basement.
- To lessen the danger of fires and explosions, follow local instructions about shutting off utility services when an attack warning sounds.
- If you have a coal-burning furnace, or a wood stove, extinguish it – or at least close all fuel and draft doors.
- Close draperies, curtains, shutters, or venetian blinds on all windows and remove furniture from window areas.

Medical Attention

Having first-aid or home-nursing skills is valuable at all times, but especially in the event of a nuclear attack. Doctors and nurses or paramedics may not be available to assist you. The survival of the injured or sick members of your family may become your responsibility. So remember to keep calm – always!

Always keep the injured person lying down in a comfortable position, head level with the body, until you determine whether the injuries are serious.

Examine a patient first for stoppage of breathing, serious bleeding, or broken bones. These must be treated *immediately*, before any attempt is made to move the injured person. Do not be hurried into moving an injured person unless you are in extreme danger.

Keep the injured person comfortably warm with blankets or other coverings, both under and over the patient.

Never attempt to give a semi-conscious or unconscious person anything to drink.

An unconscious patient lying on his back may be strangled by his own tongue, which tends to fall back and obstruct the airway. An unconscious person should be placed lying half over on his or her face (three-quarter prone position).

A patient who is breathing quietly and easily, and whose lips are pink and have no froth on them, does not have obstructed breathing. However, if the patient is breathing noisily and with difficulty, if the lips are blue and frothing, or if the patient sucks his chest inward when he breaths, the patient's airway is obstructed. *Immediate attention is needed.*

Should that be the case, place the patient on his back. Support the shoulders on a pad of any suitable material available. Tilt the head back with one hand on the forehead, the other lifting the neck. If his breathing stops, you can breathe for him by blowing air into his lungs. Take a deep breath. Pinch the patient's nostrils. Place mouth to mouth tightly. Blow into the patient's lungs strongly enough to cause his chest to rise.

This cycle should be repeated every 3 to 5 seconds for an adult, and a little more frequently for a child. Blow more gently for a child or a baby, but strongly enough to make the chest rise.

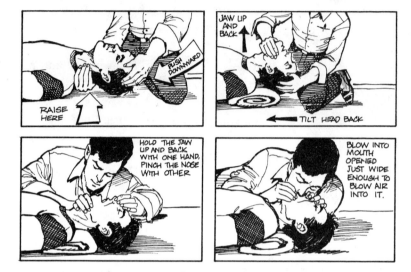

Mouth-to-mouth resuscitation is the fastest and surest way to help an unconscious person who is breathing with difficulty.

The chapter on first aid at the end of this book covers the basic treatment for wounds, burns, fractures, and other types of medical problems. But you may have problems with infant care, emotional upset, and persons suffering from radiation sickness. What to observe, and what to do for these cases, is outlined here.

INFANT CARE. Breast feeding is preferable; but if not possible, a formula using powdered or evaporated milk should be prepared under clean conditions. If vomiting or diarrhea occurs, infants and children become dehydrated very quickly. To avoid this, give frequent sips of water that has been boiled. If a rash or fever develops, keep others away from the sick child as much as may be possible within the confines of a fallout shelter.

EMOTIONAL PROBLEMS. Persons who become emotionally disturbed following a disaster should be treated calmly but firmly. They should be kept in small groups, preferably with people they know. And they should be encouraged to "talk out" their problem. If they are not otherwise injured, they should be given something to do. It may be necessary to enlist the aid of another calm person to help subdue the over-excited patient. If a stunned or dazed reaction persists for more than six to eight hours, this should be reported to a doctor or nurse as soon as one becomes available.

RADIATION SICKNESS. The signs and symptoms of this illness were described on pages 95-96. Treatment includes rest, the provision of whatever nutritious food and drink is available, and personal encouragement to get well. Swab the mouth gently with a mild, warm salt and water solution if it becomes sore. As these patients are susceptible to infection, keep wounds clean and covered with sterile dressings. Separate these patients from persons with colds, rash, or fever.

Improvised Equipment

The following suggestions may help you care for a patient when proper equipment is not available.

- bed – couch, mattress, or any well-padded, firm surface; if too low, raise on bricks, boxes, or wooden blocks.
- bedding protection – old crib pads cut into a convenient size and placed over waterproof sheeting; or several layers of newspaper and heavy brown paper covered with old soft cotton.

CAUTION

Never use thin plastic for waterproofing if the patient is a child.

- backrest – a straight-backed chair turned upside down at the head of the bed and tied securely to the bed; a triangular bolster or cushions from a chair or chesterfield.

- bed cradle – a light wooden box or firm cardboard carton, approximately 10 x 12 x 24 inches (25 x 30 x 60 centimetres), with two sides removed; or a hoop cut into two equal parts and the two pieces joined in the centre.
- pressure pads – soft cushion or foam or sponge rubber pads will protect heels, elbows, back of head, or any other body pressure point.
- bedpan (or urinal) – for bedpan, use a padded dish or pan; for urinal, use any wide-necked bottle or jar.
- hot water bottle – a heated brick wrapped in several layers of newspaper.

Emergency Cleanliness

Your limited supply of water will have to be rationed and used only for essential purposes. If you have had enough warning time before the arrival of fallout, fill your bathtub, as well as all available buckets and pans, with water and cover these receptacles.

Remember, there is an emergency supply of water in your hot-water tank.

The problems of garbage and human-waste disposal can be solved even if fallout keeps you in your shelter. Put all your garbage in tightly covered garbage pails. After using your emergency toilet, tie human waste in waterproof plastic (polyethylene) bags and place them in the garbage pail. Store a 14-day supply of bags.

After the second day in the shelter, you may risk leaving it for a few minutes for essential tasks. Therefore, when your garbage container is filled, move it out of the shelter. Keep a soft broom in the shelter for tidying up. Personal cleanliness in crowded shelter conditions is important to you and your family.

If your area is free of fallout but without sewage services, bury human waste and garbage in the ground. Dig the pit deep enough so that the waste will be covered by at least two feet of earth.

Radioactive Dust

Earlier, fallout was described as "sand." To remove the danger, remove this sand. If you suspect that your clothes have fallout on them, remove your outer clothing before going inside the house and leave the clothing outside. Don't shake those clothes inside the house or the shelter. You would only scatter the fallout grit and create unnecessary danger to others. If you have water, wash thoroughly, particularly exposed skin and hair.

CAUTION

Do not scrub your skin if you wash. This might rub in the radioactive particles.

It is important to remember that exposure to fallout *does not* make you radioactive. Even if you are stricken with radiation sickness, it is not communicable. The sickness cannot be passed on to others.

Fallout on your clothing or body would expose you and those close to you to radiation. If you suspect that you have been exposed to fallout, you will not be a danger to others if you carefully get rid of your outer clothing outside the shelter and then wash.

Since most of your food will be in tightly covered containers (cans, bottles, plastic boxes), it will all be safe to eat or drink *if* you dust the containers before opening them.

Food, if it is unspoiled and free of grit or dust, may be eaten during the emergency period. Be sure to wash fresh fruit and vegetables and then peel them carefully.

Water will be safe if it is in covered containers, or if it has come from covered wells or from undamaged water systems.

CHAPTER 9

Children and Accidents

ALL YOUNG CHILDREN get their share of cuts, bruises, and sprains in the course of growing up. Minor injuries – while upsetting at the moment – can usually be treated with a gentle swab of antiseptic, a bandage . . . and a soothing hug and kiss. Serious accidents, however, are another matter.

Normally, those who care for children want to give them all the love and protection possible. Yet, the leading cause of death and injury to young children today is accidents in the home. Why? Many people simply do not know what situations in the home can be dangerous to babies. They do not know how to avoid accidents, or how to act quickly and do the right thing when an emergency occurs.

A child is naturally active and very curious. However, a child's sense of balance and fear of danger do not develop until he matures and has some experience. An average home is full of danger for the average child: staircases, hot stoves, electric wires, and the like. All can be very dangerous to children. You cannot stop a child from being active or curious, nor would you want to. But you should create a home in which the child can safely be active. This calls for a careful, well-thought-out, and regular plan of action from you and your family.

Falls, Blows, Cuts, and Animal Bites

Severe falls are the most common form of injury to infants. But you can make your home fall-safe.

A baby is completely helpless and requires total protection. He wiggles, he rolls – you never know when he'll roll over. His crib, with the sides pulled up, and his playpen are the only safe places for the child to be left alone.

CAUTION

Never leave a child unguarded on a couch, bed, changing table, high chair, or any other high place from which he can fall.

If you have to answer the doorbell or the telephone while you're in the middle of a diaper change, wrap up the baby and take him with you or put him back in the crib. Make it a habit to take him with you if you must reach for anything that prevents you from keeping at least one protective hand on him. Turning your back, even for a second, can be risky.

Belts and any other restraining devices that come with infant equipment should be used. And make sure that all equipment your infant sits in, lies on, or plays in is stable.

High-chair trays should be properly locked. If the tray no longer locks securely, repair it or replace it. The restraining straps should always be used: they can prevent a fall during the moments when the tray is not attached. If your high chair does not have adequate safety straps, purchase a safety harness.

If the seat of the high chair seems slippery, you can make it more slip resistant by attaching rough-surfaced adhesive strips to it, such as the kind used for bathtubs.

Never allow your child to stand up in a high chair. Stay with your child while he or she is in the chair. If you have a folding high chair, be sure the locking device is secure each time you set up the chair. When a high chair is not in use, it should be put out of the way where it cannot be knocked over easily.

If the high chair is far enough away from the table or counter, your child can't push off from it.

Baby walkers, while a wonderful way to allow your child to exercise outside the playpen, can be extremely hazardous. Be sure the walker does not have exposed coil springs that can catch fingers and other body parts. Nor should there be X-shaped or other joints that can pinch or act as scissors.

A baby walker must not be able to collapse while in use. It should have a wheel base both wider and longer than the frame of the walker itself so that it will be stable and not tip. To keep the baby safe when it is using the walker, remove obstructions such as area or scatter rugs.

When your baby learns to crawl and creep – or is using a baby walker – barricade the tops and bottoms of your staircases. One of the most frequent accidents to babies at the crawling stage is falling down stairs. This is because babies learn to go *up* before they learn to go *down* safely. Inexpensive safety gates are available (avoid accordion-style gates), or you may be able to construct a barrier yourself that cannot easily be moved by a young child. Keep large toys and boxes out of the playpen if the child is unattended; these make for easy climbing and could lead to a fall.

Not only can toy boxes be used to climb on, and fall from, but they also are intriguing to enter and a child can suffocate inside. If the toy box has a hinged lid, make sure it is lightweight and has a flat inner surface. It should also have a device that will hold the lid open in a raised position. Make sure the device to hold it open is not able to pinch. It should also have ventilation holes in the lid and at least on one side near the top, so that if your child does crawl in and close the lid, he will be able to breathe. A toy box with a lid that cannot close completely would also suffice.

If made of metal, the box should not have rough or sharp edges; if made of wood, it should not have rough areas and splinters. Rounded and padded edges and corners will prevent injuries should the child fall against the box.

When your child begins to walk and climb, you will have to be extra watchful. Along with protections, you should now begin to teach about dangers. Because the toddler wants to investigate everything, windows and doors that are open are an invitation to disaster.

Keep stairs free of objects that can cause *you* to fall while carrying the baby. Avoid having extension cords and scatter rugs on the floor; if they are necessary, tape them down.

Always keep one hand free to hold the handrail on a staircase when you are carrying a child up or down the stairs. Frequently, people fall because they cannot *see* where they are going.

Be certain your hallways are well lighted and your stairways have a light fixture that can be activated from both the bottom and the top of the stairs. All rooms should have a light switch near the door so that the room can be lit without your stumbling in the dark. Night lights in hallways, bedrooms, and bathrooms are also excellent safeguards.

BATHING. A very young baby is more safely bathed in something smaller than the bathtub. Use a washbasin, the kitchen sink, a bathinette, or a small plastic tub. Use only a small amount of water at first until you get the knack of holding the baby securely. A basin or tub is less slippery if you line it with a clean diaper each time.

Hold the baby firmly so that his head is supported on your wrist, and with the fingers of that hand holding him securely in his armpit.

Bathtubs for the older child should have a non-skid bottom. You can buy inexpensive rubber mats with suction discs or adhesive on the underside. Or you can buy strips or packages of non-skid material that can be stuck in a pattern on the bottom of the tub.

CAUTION

Never leave a young child unsupervised in the bathtub, even for an instant.

GUARDING AGAINST BLOWS. Sharp-edged furniture, open drawers, and easily overturned items such as lamps, flower pots, and other heavy ornaments have been the frequent cause of severe blows to young children. Eliminate these hazards when possible. Otherwise, keep a watchful eye on your child until he is old enough to use care in not causing an accident to himself. Rounded plastic corners can be purchased to attach to sharp-cornered furniture.

If you have playground-type equipment in your yard or home, watch your child as you would at a public playground to ensure that he does not get in the way of other children's active play on swings, seesaws, and slides.

Remember, even the safest playground equipment can be involved in accidents if it is used improperly. And the equipment itself can expose a child to dangers: crushed or pinched fingers in moving parts; cuts from sharp parts and exposed screws or bolts; falls due to improper anchoring of equipment. And other hazards exist.

GUARDING AGAINST CUTS. Check around the house and remove sharp objects such as scissors, knives, razor blades, tools, and breakable objects from places your child can easily get to.

Do not allow a child to be in the yard with you if you are using a power mower. This is a dangerous piece of equipment that often tosses around stones, wires, and even broken glass and mower blades.

GUARDING AGAINST BITES. Family pets can be dangerous to very young children. Teach your child to play gently with pets and to avoid strange animals. Have your own pets properly immunized against rabies. Never leave food in bed with children. This may attract rodents and cause your child to be dangerously bitten.

Suffocation and Strangulation

The crib and playpen can sometimes be a source of grave danger to an infant. When choosing such furniture, be certain the slats on the ones you buy are spaced no more than 2 3/8 inches (6 cm) apart so the baby can't catch his head between them and strangle. Also be careful of loose slats that could come out, leaving a dangerous gap in which the baby's head could get caught.

Use bumper pads, securely tied in place. As soon as the child can stand up, set the mattress at its lowest position and lock the side rail at its highest position. Also make sure the mattress fits the crib snugly.

A baby should never sleep on or with a pillow; he might bury his head in it and suffocate.

An infant has little defence against thin, sticky plastic, such as the kind you get from the dry cleaners or the plastic wrap you use to cover food. The child's inhaling creates a suction, causing the film plastic to cling to nose and mouth, cutting off air.

CAUTION

Never use thin plastic to cover a crib mattress, and don't leave such plastic where a baby can grab it and pull it over his face.

The crib is not a playpen and should not be used as such. Nor should you continue to use a crib once the height of the side rail is less than three-quarters your child's height.

DANGEROUS TOYS AND OBJECTS. Naturally, every household has a large number of objects that are tempting to a baby in the "hands-to-mouth" stage. Before putting an infant in the playpen or on the floor to play, check the area carefully. Keep buttons, beads, pins, screws, or anything small enough to fit into the baby's mouth safely out of reach. Small objects can get lodged in the throat and cut off the child's air supply or can puncture a vital organ if swallowed.

The very first playthings a child is given – rattles – can be death-dealing. A baby can either swallow a rattle while sucking on it or fall with a rattle in its mouth, causing it to be jammed down the throat. No part or end of a rattle should be small enough to fit into your baby's mouth. Take rattles and other small objects out of the crib when the baby sleeps. Avoid these toy dangers:

• Sharp edges: Brittle plastic toys can easily be broken, exposing dangerous cutting edges. Wooden, metal, and plastic toys sometimes have sharp edges due to poor construction.

• Small parts: Tiny toys or those with small removable parts can be swallowed or become lodged in a child's windpipe, ears, or nose.

- Loud noises: Some noise-making guns and toy caps produce noise at levels that can damage hearing.
- Sharp points: Broken toys can expose dangerous prongs and knife-sharp points. Pins and staples on dolls' clothing, hair, and accessories can easily puncture an unsuspecting child. Even a stuffed toy can have barbed eyes or wired limbs that can cut or stab.
- Propelled objects: Any projectile can be used as a weapon and injure eyes in particular. Arrows or darts used by children should have non-removable rubber suction cups or protective tips such as those made of soft cork.
- Wrong toy for the wrong age: Common sense must be used both in toy selection and in play supervision. Older brothers and sisters should remember that their toys might be hazardous to their younger siblings.
- Electric toys: These must meet requirements for maximum surface temperatures and electrical construction, and must bear prominent warning labels. Toys that include heating elements are recommended only for children older than eight, but that does not mean that every eight-year-old is mature enough to use such a toy. The misuse of even safe electric toys can cause shocks or burns. Electric toys should be used cautiously under adult supervision.

CAUTION

Toys damaged beyond repair should be discarded immediately.

The most dangerous toys for a child under the age of three are those small enough to swallow. Don't let a young child play with marbles, small plastic toys, toys with easily detachable pieces, or stuffed animals and dolls with tiny button eyes or ornaments that the child can easily pull off.

Never allow the child to suck or chew on balloons.

Tricycles are another danger potential. If you are getting a tricycle for your child, make sure it's the right size. For extra stability, it should be low slung with the seat close to the ground and the wheels widely spaced. The pedals and hand-grips should have rough, non-slip surfaces.

Safe riding habits should be taught before the tricycle is used. Caution children against riding double and remind them that the moving spokes on the wheels are dangerous traps for feet and hands. Riding down hills is dangerous because tricycles do not have brakes.

Don't feed a very young child popcorn, nuts, or small hard candies. Young children do not know how to eat these properly and they can easily get inhaled into the windpipe instead of going to the stomach. The same warning applies to pills. Use liquid medication or crushed and diluted pills.

Abandoned refrigerators and trunks are very dangerous. Children love to play and hide in them. Suffocation easily results. Remove doors from refrigerators and lids from trunks.

Poisoning

Fatal poisonings are most frequent in children between the ages of one and three. Some doctors refer to this stage in a child's development as "The Age of Accidents." Children often explore by tasting things *and will eat and drink anything they find, no matter how bad it may taste*. To protect your child against possible poisoning, you should:

- Know which substances in and around your home are poisonous.
- Keep those poisons out of your child's reach at all times.
- Never underestimate your child's cleverness and skill at getting to poisons.

If you don't know what substances around the home are poisonous, you should be aware that nearly all household chemicals and drugs contain poisonous elements. Look for manufacturers' warnings on the labels of products you bring home. These may read as follows: "Poison," "Caution: Harmful if Swallowed," "For External Use Only," "Keep Out of the Reach of Children." Now inspect your home carefully and see how many of the products you have around bear such warnings. Be certain such poisons are kept out of your child's reach at all times. Here are some of the poisonous items that are frequently found in most households.

- ASA (Aspirin) and other medications
- Insect repellants and rat poisons
- Kerosene, gasoline, turpentine, benzine, and any cleaning fluid
- Furniture and automobile polish
- Lye and other alkalis used for cleaning drains, toilet bowls, and ovens
- Oil of wintergreen
- Plant sprays
- Bleach, ammonia, washing soda, and detergents
- Mothballs

Unmarked Poisons

You cannot entirely rely on a product label to give you the proper warning at all times. Poisonous items such as nail polish, perfume, cosmetics, and hair tonics may offer no clue as to the hazards of accidental swallowing. Prescription drugs and some over-the-counter medicines do not carry warnings about the dangers of overdose or accidental swallowing.

Alcoholic beverages, such as gin, whisky, beer, and wine, are sold in containers that have no cautionary wording about the harm they can cause a child who might drink large quantities of the contents.

Since you can't possibly know which of the hundreds of varieties of these medicines, cosmetics, and general household products are potentially dangerous, your best line of defence is to suspect anything that is not a known and healthy food item.

Poisonous Plants

A surprising number of house plants are capable of poisoning. While the plant that the child nibbled at may supposedly have been harmless – even though you find the child's tongue is swelling, his mouth is afire, and he's crying – you must check with your local poison-control centre or your doctor immediately. The plants that are most dangerous are:

DIEFFENBACHIA. These plants cause an irritation to the skin or mouth. The sensation is a little like "tiny needles in the mouth." Eating leaves from these plants is rarely fatal, but a problem can develop with respiration if the throat swells. The immediate antidote for poisoning from *dieffenbachia, philodendron,* or *dumb cane* is something cool and soothing with lots of calcium – like milk, ice cream, or yogurt.

HYACINTH, NARCISSUS. The toxic part of these plants is the bulb, which looks a bit like an onion. Nibbling on these can cause nausea or vomiting.

OLEANDER. This plant contains a cardiac drug similar to digitalis that can slow down the heart rate. The danger depends on the season and the parts of the plant the child has ingested. An intestinal upset is usually the first manifestation of the problem.

CASTOR BEANS, ROSARY PEAS. While these are not common houseplants, the seeds can be found in jewelry manufactured in Third World countries. A string of beads can break and the child will eat one. The beans cause severe irritation to the intestinal tract.

POINSETTIA. Toxic, but a child would have to swallow a pound of leaves to become seriously ill.

Other household plants that may cause problems are *daffodils* and *elephant ear.* Of course, household plants are not the only villains in the green world. Certain plants, shrubs, and trees in your garden can cause problems. The outdoor list includes the following:

Flowers

Larkspur	Star of Bethlehem	Autumn Crocus
Monkshood	Lily of the Valley	Irish Foxglove
Bleeding Heart		

Ornamental Shrubs

Daphne	Rhododendron	Golden Chain
Wisteria	Jessamine	Azalea
Laurel	Lantan camara (red sage)	Yew

Trees and Shrubs

Wild and cultivated cherry	Black Locust
Elderberry	Oak

Field Plants

Buttercups   Nightshade   Poison hemlock   Jimson Weed

Plants in Wooded Areas

Jack-in-the-pulpit   Moonseed   Mayapple

Vegetables

Rhubarb leaves

Even nibbling on leaves, sucking on plant stalks, and drinking water in which plants have been soaking may cause poisoning.

Food Poisoning

Proper sterilization of a baby's formula and prompt refrigeration of milk and opened jars of baby food are extremely important habits to form to prevent the growth of harmful bacteria that can cause food poisoning.

Some non-poisonous food substances can be just as dangerous as poisonous ones when given to an infant by mistake – for example, putting salt instead of sugar into a baby's formula. If you transfer items such as salt and sugar into other containers, be sure you label the new containers – and read the label before using the contents.

Medicine

When giving any medication, always follow the directions on the label or, in the case of prescription drugs, the doctor's instructions. Never make the mistake of thinking: "If a little medicine is good, a lot is better."

An overdose of good-tasting medicine is one of the leading causes of poisoning in young children. Children love the taste of such medicines and will climb to great heights to search for them, especially if they are hungry. *Never* encourage your child to take medicine by telling him that it is "candy." Such misinformation has often encouraged children to search for these medicines and swallow huge and dangerous quantities of them.

CAUTION

Candy-flavoured Aspirin and vitamin tablets tempt some children to search for them. If you use these products, find a good hiding place for them – or better yet, lock them up.

Lead Poisoning

A great deal has been written about the dangers of lead poisoning to young children. The main source of lead poisoning in the home is dried, peeling paint on walls, woodwork, repainted furniture, and repainted toys.

Children suck and chew on toys and furniture all the time. They will pick at peeling paint and loose plaster until they pull off a piece – and into the mouth it goes! If you repaint anything inside your house use only unaltered lead-free paint.

Even if you do paint with a lead-free paint, there may be layers of old paint underneath that have a high lead content. Take no chances: scrape off *all* layers of old and peeling paint. Wrap up the scrapings, tie the package securely, and dispose of it outside in a covered container.

When your child is outdoors, however, you will have to have a watchful eye. Most outdoor paints do have a high lead content. Do not let your child bite down on window sills, porch steps, or bars on iron fences and gates.

Some infants display an unusual appetite for inedible substances such as paint chips, plaster, crayons, chalk, wallpaper, dirt, and cigarettes. This abnormal craving is called "pica." A child with this malady must be well protected, for persistent pica can cause lead poisoning. If your child shows these symptoms, it would be wise to talk the problem over with a doctor.

It is impossible not to have poisonous substances around the house, therefore it is essential to know where to keep them. Here are six general rules to follow:

- Never keep household cleaners and chemicals under the sink or on low-lying shelves where your crawling or toddling child can easily find them and be tempted to sample their contents. Store these items in a high cabinet, preferably one that can be locked.
- Dispose of empty poison containers in a safe receptacle *outside* the house where the child can't fish them out and play with them.
- Always remember to put medicine and household chemicals away *immediately* after using them. If the phone rings or you go to answer the door while you're using medicine or a chemical, take the bottle with you. Don't turn your back on a child while a poisonous substance is within his reach.
- Do not underestimate a child's cleverness and skill in getting to poisons. Children will display skills that parents never dream they have yet developed – opening doors, unscrewing bottle caps (sometimes even so-called child-proof caps), squeezing bottles, opening purses, and even remembering where poisonous substances are kept.
- Don't transfer potential poisons into food containers such as bowls, jars, or soft drink or milk bottles. Many people do this, especially when using kerosene, turpentine, spot remover, or bleach. Youngsters innocently identify the container with a familiar drink and sometimes swallow its contents before parents can stop them.
- Poisonous substances should *never* be stored around foods. Adults have also mistaken such poisons as roach powder and boric acid solutions for food and have caused fatal poisoning.

Drowning

Never leave your child alone in the bathtub, wading pool, or around open or frozen bodies of water. Drowning only takes seconds, and even shallow water is dangerous.

Do not leave your bathtub filled or leave tubs of water or wading pools where a baby can fall into them. As a rule, expect a child to seek out interesting water in the neighbourhood – a swimming pool, storm sewers, wading pool, or whatever. Make certain such areas are securely fenced off or supervised.

Fires, Burns, and Electric Shock

Chapters One and Two of this book cover the hazards of fire and electricity. Therefore, the problems as they pertain to children are only briefly touched on here.

Every year a startling number of babies and young children die or are injured in fires. Careless smoking and children playing with matches and lighters cause one out of every five fires. Don't tempt children by leaving matches and lighters around.

Never leave a child alone in a house. In minutes he could kindle a fire, or one could spring up and trap him. Children panic easily in fires and, when parents are not there to rescue them, they have been known to do foolish things such as hide under beds or in closets.

Home fire-drills are an excellent safety measure. The best way to avoid panic in case of fire is to know what you are going to do *before* a fire ever breaks out.

Your first impulse in a fire should always be *escape*. Too many people become unnecessary fire victims because they underestimate the killing power and speed of fire. If the fire is very small and has just started, you can possibly extinguish it yourself with the proper equipment at hand. (See chart on page 24.)

CAUTION

In the event of a fire, you must always get children outside first.

Smoke, not flames, is the real killer in a fire. According to some studies, as many as 80 per cent of deaths are due to inhaling poisonous fumes long before the flames ever came near the person.

Preventing Burns

Fireplaces, open heaters, hot registers, floor furnaces, and radiators all have caused horrible burns to babies. Since you cannot watch your child all the time, you should screen fireplaces and put guards around heaters, furnaces, registers, and radiators.

Sometimes you may have to use a vapourizer or portable heater in the baby's room. Be sure it is located beyond the child's hand reach, and do not place it close to the child's bedclothes.

Use caution in the kitchen. It is not safe to let an infant crawl, or a small child walk, around the kitchen while you are cooking or serving meals. There is danger of your tripping and spilling something hot on the baby, or of spattering grease on him, or even of the child pulling a hot pot off the stove onto himself.

This is the best time for the playpen or high chair. Even then, be certain the baby's chair or playpen is well away from the stove. Get into the habit of always turning pot handles inward toward the back of the stove and never leaving the oven door open. Avoid tablecloths that hang over the table's edge. The child may grasp the cloth and pull hot foods down on himself.

Preventing Electric Shock

It is easier to prevent electric shock than it is to treat it. To a child, an electric outlet is a fascinating hole in the wall, just right for poking. Use child-proof covers on unused electric outlets to keep out the baby's fingers and toys or other objects. To further safeguard against shock, have damaged appliances and frayed cords repaired promptly. A defect can produce a lethal jolt. Certainly never let a child play with or chew on an electric cord.

If your child receives an electric shock, the first thing to do is to see *if he is still in contact with the live wire*.

If the child is NOT CONNECTED to the wire: 1. Give him artificial respiration immediately. The electric shock stops the victim's respiration and sometimes his heart. 2. Treat his burns as soon as possible. The electric spark can cause a severe burn. 3. Call a doctor (or, if possible, have someone else call the doctor while you are treating the child).

If the child IS CONNECTED to the wire, do not try to pull him away with your bare hands. You may get a severe shock yourself and that won't do you or the child any good. Shut off the current, preferably at the main switch. If that should prove difficult – for any one of a variety of reasons – then remove the extension cord from the wall socket. Should that prove impossible for any reason, you must pull the live wire away from the child. But *remember* to use a dry stick or rubber gloves or a rolled, or folded, piece of newspaper to move the wire.

If you have to pull the child away while he is still touching the wire, *do not* touch the child with your bare hands. Use

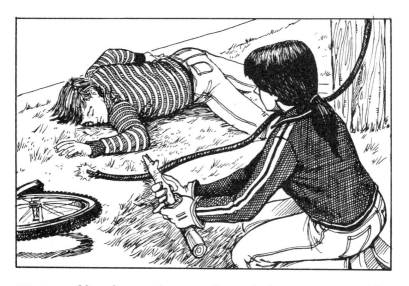

Wearing rubber gloves and using a dry stick, the rescuer is carefully moving a live wire away from an electric-shock victim.

rubber gloves, or heavy cloth gloves (like oven mitts), folds of cloth or paper, or a wooden pole or board – anything that is not made of metal and is dry. Then give the child artificial respiration and first aid – and call a doctor.

Be Prepared for an Emergency

Even after you have done everything you can think of to protect your child from accidents, they can still happen.

In an emergency, the most important advice can also be the most difficult to follow if you are not prepared. That is:

Keep calm – do not panic.

CHAPTER **10**

Hazards Away from Home

BEING AWAY FROM HOME can be as hazardous as being at home – or more so. Many people are unaware of the hazards that can face them when they are "on the road." Within the security of your car, you can be exposed to many dangers. When you're on the streets or out shopping, or on a trip – whether it's for business or pleasure – or even when you're at your place of work, there are hazards that you can help prevent, or at least alleviate, if you are prepared for them.

Fear is a normal reaction for everyone facing an emergency that threatens any of his or her important needs. But fear may ruin your chances for coping successfully with an emergency, or it could actually improve them.

There is no advantage to denying fear or the existence of danger. There is usually something that can be done to improve the situation. Acceptance of fear as a natural reaction to a threatening situation will lead to purposeful rather than panicky behaviour and will greatly increase chances for survival.

Fear must be recognized, lived with, and, if possible, utilized to advantage. Factors increasing fear are mainly helplessness and hopelessness. One of the fear-reducing factors most frequently reported by people who have faced unexpected emergencies was *concentrating on the job to be done*.

In Case of Fire

For the person who travels the fear of fire in his home-away-from-home, the hotel, can be overpowering. Most hotels have installed a variety of systems to warn the guest in case of fire and to assist in safe evacuation if that becomes necessary.

Panic often leads people to do things that are fatal: run toward a fire rather than away from it; crowd into overloaded elevators instead of walking down fireproof stairwells; jump from windows or roofs when help is at hand. It is important, therefore, to know what you are going to do and where you will be going in the event of a fire in your hotel.

As has been pointed out in earlier chapters, most people who are killed in fires die of smoke inhalation. Even a very small fire can produce a great deal of smoke – and worse, great quantities of toxic gases. In fact, the ventilation systems in large buildings such as hotels tend to carry the smoke and gases from room to room, transmitting them far from the actual flames. In that way, the oxygen supply in your room can be displaced very quickly, even though the flames themselves are not even close.

As soon as you check into a hotel and put your luggage in your room, check the floor map on the back of the room door. Then go back into the hall (remembering to take your key with you and lock your door!) and find the fire exit. Count the number of doors between your room and the fire exit. Note turns in the hall. You do all this so that you can make a mental map and be able, in the event of an emergency, to find that fire exit in the dark, or through smoke-filled halls, or even with your eyes closed (smoke and gases could irritate the membranes of the eyes and force them tightly shut).

When you go to sleep at night or take a nap, put your room key where you can get it easily – and always in the same place. Then, if you decide to leave your room in the event of fire, you can find your key quickly and *take it with you*.

If the door to your room is not of the self-closing variety, remember to close it after you. If the passage to the exit is blocked by fire and smoke, you will want to return to your room and await help. Having had the foresight to take your key, you can now get back in.

Should you leave your room in the event of a fire, or should you not? Touch the inside of the door. If it is very hot, *do not* open it. The fire could be right outside your door or might be in a place that would block your escape route. So stay where you are and plan on your next actions to protect yourself until help arrives.

1. If the telephone is working, call the desk and alert them to your situation.
2. If the windows can be opened, open them to vent the smoke.

CAUTION

Do not break hotel windows if they don't open. You may find smoke pouring into your room from the outside. You may also cut yourself.

3. Fill the bathtub with water. Scoop out buckets of water – using the ice bucket or waste basket – and soak the door and walls to cool them. Then soak sheets and towels, and stuff them in the cracks around the door to keep smoke out of the room.
4. If smoke is seeping into your room, tie a wet hand towel over your nose and mouth to filter the air you breathe.

If, however, the door is cool to your touch, you can take your key and check the halls and the route to the fire exit that you investigated earlier. If there is smoke in the halls, crawl along the escape route. Smoke is hot and therefore rises, so the air next to the floor should be fresher and safer to breathe.

Remain against the wall on which the fire exit is located. Count the doors until you reach the fire door. When you reach the stairwell, walk – *don't run* – down the stairs. Hold firmly to the handrail because others escaping may panic and push, and you could lose your footing.

On the way down, if you should suddenly encounter thick smoke, *do not* try to get through. Walk back up. If the fire door doesn't open to let you back onto your floor, continue to the roof. Prop the door open and move to the windward side of the building.

CAUTION

Never leave a high-rise building by taking the elevator. It could prove a fatal trap for a variety of reasons.

If, while staying in a hotel, you should smell smoke or suspect fire, immediately call the switchboard operator. Don't be deterred if the line is busy; the switchboard may be loaded with similar calls. Don't panic: decide whether you will try to leave as described above, or wait a few minutes to try the phone again to get a report or instructions.

Safety in Your Car

As you might in your home, you feel a certain amount of security when you are in your own automobile. But the hazards can be even greater in the car than in the home. The same troubles you can experience at home can be experienced in the car: theft, fire, accident.

Cars are susceptible to break-and-enter, therefore they are not satisfactory places to protect valuables. In addition, the car itself holds attractions of its own for the burglar – radio and tape player, for example. Tires, hubcaps, and rims can be sold to junk dealers and can be removed far too simply. The car itself is a tempting invitation to a thief.

So before you enter your car look around. Are any of the tires flat? Are there obstructions in front of any of the wheels? Is there any sign of tampering with the door handles or other attempts at break-in? If anything seems unnatural or disturbed, walk away and phone the police. If everything seems to be in order, unlock the door – assuming that you locked it when you left the car. If you did, and the door is now unlocked, be wary. Check to see if your car radio and tape deck are there and if the glove compartment has not been disturbed. If the car doesn't start, lock the car and seek help as quickly and carefully as possible. Any stranger who suddenly appears and tries to force his assistance on you should be considered with extreme suspicion.

The same applies to strangers who seek assistance – especially on a lonely stretch of highway. You might stop and roll down your window just enough to talk and to determine the nature of the problem, then go for assistance. To do anything else may be very risky.

Winter Travel

Travelling in your car during the winter months can be a serious business. If you do a lot of winter driving, you should consider two things:
• Joining the Canadian Automobile Association.
• Installing a Citizen's Band radio.

The hazards of winter driving fall into five major categories:

BLIZZARD. This is the most perilous of winter storms, combining snow that is falling, blowing, and drifting with winds of 25 miles an hour (40 km/h) or more. The conditions make for poor visibility and are accompanied by low temperatures made more dangerous by the wind-chill factor. A blizzard is likely to last six or more hours.

HEAVY SNOW. When the snow falls at the rate of four inches (10 cm) or more in 12 hours, or six inches (15 cm) or more in 24 hours it is considered a heavy fall in snow country. In more temperate climates, less snowfall than that is considered heavy.

FREEZING RAIN OR DRIZZLE. This is an ice storm that coats roads, trees, overhead wires, etc., with ice.

COLD WAVE. A rapid fall in temperature in a short period calls for greater than normal protective measures.

WINDS. These cause blizzard conditions, drifting, reduced visibility, and wind-chill effects.

Always heed the warnings. Local weather offices of the atmospheric environment services issue warnings on weather conditions for all the hazards of winter.

When winter approaches, make sure that you take your car in for a winter checkup. This should include your ignition system, battery, lights, cooling system, fuel system, lubrication, exhaust system, heater, brakes, wipers, defroster, snow tires, chains, antifreeze, and winter oil.

If you do any amount of country driving in the winter months, keep a winter storm-kit in your trunk. Even for city driving you should have some of these items with you:

Shovel	Emergency food	Ice scraper and
Tow chain	pack	brush
Compass	Road maps	Flashlight
Sand	Booster cables	Extra clothing and
Warning light	Axe or hatchet	footwear
or road flares	First-aid kit	Methyl hydrate
Matches	Blanket	(for fuel line
Fire	Candle in deep	and windshield
extinguisher	can	de-icing)

If you must travel in winter conditions there are six rules you should heed:
- Drive with caution. Adjust your speed to road conditions and drive defensively.
- Don't press on. If the going gets tough, turn back or seek refuge.
- Try to keep to main roads.
- Make sure you have ample gasoline.
- Keep your radio tuned to a local station for weather advice.
- Above all, don't take unnecessary risks.

If You Get Trapped

The first thing you must remember is *not to panic*. Avoid over-exertion and exposure. Stay in your car: you won't get lost and you will have shelter.

Keep fresh air in your car. Open a lee-side window. Run your engine sparingly. Beware of exhaust fumes. To assure that no exhaust fumes are getting into the car, check to see that drifting snow has not blocked your exhaust pipe.

Set out a warning light or flares. Turn on the dome light.

Limit or avoid use of your headlights lest you run your battery down. Exercise your limbs, hands, and feet vigorously. Keep moving and keep watch for traffic and searchers.

CAUTION

If trapped in your car in a winter storm, it is essential that you do not fall asleep.

Other Hazards of Winter

Too many people are unaware of the hazards of winter. Harsh conditions of wind, cold snow, or whiteout can turn an outing into a tragedy. Knowledge of the area, weather, route, and the limitations of your body and equipment, plus some common sense, can ensure safe and enjoyable outings.

Before you leave, notify a responsible person of your planned route of travel. Mark it on a map. Give your planned time of departure and return. And immediately upon your return, check with that person.

Plan on clothing that can be layered so that you can adjust what you are wearing to prevailing conditions. A good-quality windbreaking jacket and wind pants are essential.

Avoid tight-fitting clothes and boots that may restrict circulation. Take extra socks and gloves or mittens, as well as a toque or balaclava.

In your emergency kit have matches in a waterproof container, candle, fire-starter (000 steel wool works well when pulled apart), nylon cord, general-purpose knife, high-energy food, plastic tarp, space blanket, signal mirror, first-aid kit, wide tape for repairs, and a metal container in which you can melt snow.

If you're using a snowmobile for transportation, make sure that you have the appropriate tools for repairs, as well as extra spark plugs and drive belt. Experienced snowmobilers always carry snowshoes in the event of machine failure, in addition to the normal emergency and survival gear listed in the previous paragraph.

As for food and water, the best rule is "lightweight but loaded," meaning loaded with calories. Plan your meals to ensure a diet of high-energy foods. Water is often difficult to find in winter; all that may be available is what you have carried with you or can melt from snow in the metal container you have for that purpose. Remember that the body loses as much as two to four quarts (two to four litres) of fluid daily under exertion. This must be replaced in order for you to maintain good physical condition.

Eating snow provides only limited water (10 to 20 per cent of snow is water, the rest is air). But more important, it drains energy from the body, which has to expend heat to melt the snow, and thereby body temperature is cooled. Avoid melting snow by body contact for the same reason – it lowers your body temperature quickly, and you must save your energy. Therefore, be equipped to melt snow.

Recreational Hazards

Large and small snow avalanches can have tremendous force and are a serious threat to the skier, snowmobiler, snowshoer, or other person who enjoys snow sports. Understanding the basic types of avalanches as well as understanding the contributions of terrain and weather factors, along with carefully selecting a safe route, can help you avoid being caught in this kind of natural disaster. It will also help you survive if you are buried in one.

Snow avalanches are complex natural phenomena. Experts do not fully understand all their underlying causes. It is difficult to predict avalanche conditions with certainty, but you can develop judgement about the presence and degree of avalanche danger. There are two principal types of snow avalanches: *loose snow* and *slab*.

Loose snow avalanches start at one point or over a small area. They grow in size and the amount of snow involved increases as the avalanche descends. Loose snow moves as a formless mass with little internal cohesion.

Slab avalanches, on the other hand, start when a large area of snow begins to slide at once. There is a well-defined fracture line where the snow breaks away, and these avalanches are characterized by the tendency of snow crystals to stick together. There may be angular blocks or chunks of snow in the slide.

The latter type are responsible for most accidents. Many times the victims have triggered the avalanche themselves. Their weight on the stressed snow is enough to break the fragile bonds that hold it to the slope.

There are obviously many factors that affect snow avalanches: the steepness of the slope, its convexness, and the way it faces (north-facing slopes are dangerous in winter, south-facing ones in spring and on sunny days). Ground cover can help anchor the snow, though avalanches have been known to start among trees. Weather plays its part: temperature, wind, storms, rate of snowfall, and type of snow on the ground.

If you are caught in an avalanche, these actions are essential to survival:
• Discard all equipment.
• If you're on a snowmobile, get away from it.
• Make swimming motions as the snow surrounds you. Try to stay on top and work your way to the side of the downflow.
• Before coming to a stop, try to make an air pocket in front of your face with your hands.
• Remain calm.

If you are in a party and are the only survivor, mark the place you last saw victims. Search directly downslope beyond the point you last saw the others in your party and if they are not on the surface, scuff or probe the snow with a pole or stick.

CAUTION

Do not desert the victims in an avalanche by going for help, unless help is only a few minutes away. After 30 minutes, the buried victim has only a 50 per cent chance of surviving.

If there is more than one survivor, send one for help while the others search for victims. Make sure the help-seeker marks the route so the rescue party can find its way to the scene.

Hypothermia

The number-one killer of outdoor recreationists is hypothermia – subnormal body temperature. Lowering of internal temperature leads to mental and physical collapse. Hypothermia is caused by exposure to cold, and it is aggravated by wetness, wind, and exhaustion.

Cold kills in two distinct steps. The first is exposure and exhaustion. The moment you begin to lose heat faster than your body produces it, you are undergoing exposure. Two things happen: you voluntarily exercise to stay warm; and your body makes involuntary adjustments to preserve normal temperature in its vital organs. Both responses drain your energy reserves. The only way to stop the drain is to reduce the degree of exposure.

The second step is hypothermia. If the exposure continues until your energy reserves are exhausted, cold reaches the brain, depriving you of judgement and reasoning power. You will not be aware this is happening. You will lose control of your hands. This is the first indication of hypothermia. Your internal temperature is sliding downward and this slide, without treatment, leads to stupor, collapse, and death.

Remember, the time to prevent hypothermia is during the period of exposure and gradual exhaustion.

What defences do you have against this killer?

• Stay dry. When your clothes get wet, they lose about 90 per cent of their insulating value. Wool loses less; cotton, synthetics, and down lose more. Choose clothes that are waterproof against wind-driven rain, and cover head, neck, body, and legs. Polyurethane-coated nylon is best. But the coating doesn't last forever, so in.spect the coat carefully and test it under a cold shower before you leave home. Ponchos are poor protection from the wind.

- Beware of the wind. A slight breeze carries heat away from bare skin much faster than still air. Wind drives cold air under and through clothing. Wind refrigerates wet clothes by evaporating moisture from the surface. Wind multiplies the problems of staying dry. Take woollen clothing for hypothermia weather. Include a knit toque or balaclava that can protect neck and chin. Remember that cotton underwear is worse than useless when wet.

- Understand cold. Most hypothermia cases develop in air temperatures between 32° and 50°F (0° and 10°C). Many outdoorsmen can't believe that above-freezing temperatures can be dangerous. They underestimate the danger of being wet when it's that cold – with fatal results.Water at 50°F (10°C) is unbearably cold. The cold that kills is cold water running down neck and legs, cold water held against the body by sopping wet clothes, and cold water flushing body heat from the surface of the clothes.

- Use your clothes. Put on raingear *before* you get wet. Put on wool clothing *before* you start to shiver.

- End exposure. If you cannot stay warm and dry under existing weather conditions by using the clothes you have with you, then end your exposure. Be smart enough to give up reaching that mountain peak or catching that long-elusive fish or whatever it was you had in mind.

- Get out of the wind and rain. Build a fire. Concentrate on making your camp or bivouac as secure and comfortable as possible.

CAUTION

Do not ignore shivering. Persistent or violent shivering is clear warning that you are on the verge of hypothermia.

Keep nibbling trail foods (nuts, jerky, candy) during hypothermia weather. Having chosen your outdoors equipment with hypothermia in mind, make camp while you still have a reserve of energy. Allow for the fact that exposure greatly reduces your normal endurance. And exercise will drain your energy reserves.

If exhaustion forces you to stop, your body heat production instantly drops 50 per cent or more. Violent, incapacitating shivering may begin immediately, and you may slip into hypothermia in a matter of minutes.

If your party is exposed to wind, cold, and wet, *think hypothermia*. Watch yourself and others for these symptoms.
• Uncontrollable fits of shivering.
• Vague, slow, slurred speech.
• Memory lapses, incoherence.
• Frequent stumbling and lurching gait.
• Immobile, fumbling hands.
• Apparent exhaustion; inability to get up after a rest.
• Drowsiness. Remember, *to sleep is to die*.

The victim may deny he's in trouble. *Believe the symptoms, not the victim*. Even mild symptoms demand immediate, drastic treatment.
1. Get the victim out of the wind and rain.
2. Strip off all his wet clothes.
3. If the victim is only mildly impaired, give him warm drinks, warm clothing, and a warm sleeping bag. Well-wrapped, warm (not hot) rocks or canteens will hasten recovery.
4. If the victim is semiconscious or worse, try to keep him awake. Give him warm drinks. Leave him stripped and put him into a sleeping bag with another person, who also is stripped. If you have a double bag, put the victim between two warmth donors. Skin-to-skin contact is the most effective treatment.
5. Build a fire to warm the camp.

Other Dangers

There are five other problem areas you can encounter in winter activities. These are wind-chill factor, dehydration, frostbite, altitude sickness, and hyperventilation.

Wind Chill

Wind, temperature, and moisture are factors that can greatly affect the safety of the winter traveller or sports enthusiast. Each contributes to the loss of body heat. Wind and temperature will affect a dry, properly clothed person. If clothing is wet from perspiration or precipitation, however, the net effect of wind and temperature is all the greater. This effect is very difficult for many people to understand because there isn't a convenient "meter" to measure the wind chill as there is to measure temperature and humidity. Your best bet is to realize that the stronger the wind, the more you are affected by the wind-chill factor.

Wind can, for example, produce the equivalent of a temperature of 0°F (-18°C) when the actual temperature is only at 32°F (0°C) and the wind is blowing at 25 miles an hour (40 km/h). In other words, when the thermometer reads at the freezing point, a modest wind drops the wind-chill factor to an uncomfortable situation.

Dehydration

Even if you are inactive, as an adult you require two quarts (about two litres) of water daily. Twice as much is needed by your body if you are engaged in strenuous activity. Should you lose three pints (1.5 litres) of water from your body, you will suffer a 25 per cent loss of stamina. Therefore, to avoid dehydration, simply drink as often as you feel thirsty.

Frostbite

If your flesh is inadequately protected against subfreezing temperatures, frostbite can result. Tissue damage is caused by the reduced blood flow to the extremities – as opposed to hypothermia, which causes lowering of the body's rate of metabolism. Your skin takes on a dead white appearance and you suffer a loss of feeling. Should this happen, you must restore body temperature as rapidly as possible, preferably by immersion in a water bath of less than 110°F (30°C), or by other means. If it is necessary to keep moving, then keep the affected part covered and move the victim to a location where effective treatment and evacuation by vehicle can be obtained.

When you are out in a party, periodically observe your companions (especially their noses and cheeks) for signs of frostbite.

Remember, if you're on a snowmobile you will be especially susceptible to frostbite because of the speed at which the wind moves past you.

Altitude Sickness

At 10,000 feet (3,000 metres), air contains only two-thirds of the volume of oxygen that it does at sea level. In addition, the higher air pressure at sea level easily forces the available oxygen through the thin lining of the lungs into the bloodstream. At higher elevations there is less air pressure and the available oxygen is not so easily forced through the lung walls.

If the altitude starts to affect you, you will become listless and lose your appetite. Weakness, apathy, nausea, dizziness, and drowsiness also develop. The minute you sense any of these symptoms, stop and rest. Breathe deeply a few times, then take some nourishment that is high in sugar content: candy, fruit juices, or even sugar itself. Move back to lower elevations.

The best way to prevent altitude sickness is to keep in good physical condition and maintain a well-balanced diet. Avoid trips to high altitudes that may immediately involve physical exercise.

Hyperventilation

This is a reaction to altitude caused by too rapid breathing and decrease of the carbon dioxide level in the blood. The result is lightheadedness and a cold feeling. The victim usually becomes apprehensive and excited. Therefore, the first thing to do is to calm the victim, have him relax, and make him breathe into a flexible container – such as a glove, paper bag, or hat – until normal breathing is restored.

Again, being in good physical condition and maintaining good dietary habits should prevent hyperventilation. And sudden trips to high places that will involve immediate physical activity should be avoided.

First Aid: A Survival Guide

WHAT SHOULD YOU DO if a family member is suddenly injured or becomes ill? Right after an accident or a sudden serious illness occurs, and before professional medical help can take over, there is a critical period in which the availability of a person skilled in first-aid techniques can mean the difference between life and death.

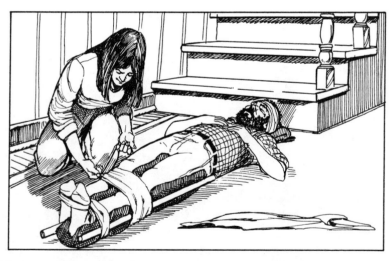

Making the victim immobile will prevent possible complications of leg injuries after an accident.

First aid does not replace the physician; it does attempt to keep the victim alive and in the best condition possible until medical aid arrives. And, of course, there are also minor injuries that, if improperly treated, can become serious problems.

When a person becomes injured or ill, someone must take charge, send for a doctor if necessary, and apply first aid. The person taking charge must make a quick but adequate examination to determine the nature of the injuries.

CAUTION

Never move an injured person until you have a clear idea of the injury and have applied first aid, unless the victim is exposed to further danger at the injury site.

If the injury is serious, if it occurred in an area where the victim can remain safely, and if medical help is readily obtainable, it is best not to move the victim but to employ such emergency care as is possible at the site until qualified emergency personnel arrive.

In making your initial survey prior to administering first aid, observe the victim carefully, listen to what he tells you (if he is conscious), and if there were other witnesses to the accident ask them what they saw.

In other words, *make no assumptions*. The obvious injuries may not be the only ones present. Less noticeable injuries may also have occurred. You should also look for causes of the injury – this may provide a clue as to the extent of the physical damage.

While there are several conditions that can be considered life-threatening, *respiratory arrest* and *severe bleeding* require attention first. Only when these problems have been alleviated should attention be focused on other obvious injuries: open chest or abdominal wounds should be sealed, open fractures immobilized, burns covered, and less serious bleeding wounds dressed.

Remember always to handle the victim carefully. Any unnecessary movement or rough handling might aggravate undetected fractures, spinal injuries, or internal injuries.

In an emergency, seconds and minutes can make the difference between life and death. Decisive, quick, and proper action by you can save a life.

The Call for Help

If an injured person is in distress but breathing, call for emergency assistance at once. If the victim is *not* breathing, help him first and call later. Or get someone else to call while you are trying to resuscitate the victim. This is the information you should provide when you reach emergency service:

1. Give the phone number from which you are calling.
2. Give the address and any special directions on how to get to the accident scene.
3. Describe the victim's condition in the best fashion you can: burned, bleeding, broken bones, etc.
4. Give your name.

CAUTION

Do not hang up on an emergency call. Let the emergency services people terminate the conversation. They may have questions to ask or special information to give you about what you can do until help arrives.

Life-Threatening Conditions

There are four life-threatening conditions that have to be attended to before any other first-aid treatment is given. These are:

• Impaired breathing
• Circulatory failure
• Severe bleeding
• Shock

Obviously, immediate recognition and correction of these conditions is of first and paramount concern. Emergency treatment should be given in this order, as necessary:

1. Clear the air passage.

2. Restore breathing and heartbeat.
3. Stop bleeding.
4. Administer treatment for shock.

Impaired Breathing

The causes of impaired breathing can be any of the following:
• Suffocation
• Gas poisoning
• Electric shock
• Drowning
• Heart failure

The signs and symptoms will be:
• The chest or abdomen does not rise and fall.
• Air cannot be felt exiting from the nose or mouth.

FIRST-AID TREATMENT. There are several methods of artificial respiration. Mouth-to-mouth is the most effective. Use the mouth-to-nose method if the victim has a severe jaw fracture or mouth wound, or has his jaws tightly closed. Simply breathe into his nose instead of his mouth. (See **Artificial Respiration**.)

Use the manual method only when mouth-to-mouth cannot be used: for example, if the victim has severe facial injuries or is trapped or pinned face down.

Remember, seconds count when a person is not breathing. Start artificial respiration at once. Don't take time to move the victim unless the accident site remains unsafe.

Breathing may be impaired by a foreign object stuck in the victim's throat. The signs or symptoms in such an event are:
• The victim gasps for breath.
• The victim may have violent fits of coughing.
• The victim turns pale, then blue . . . quickly.
• The victim cannot talk or breathe.

FIRST-AID TREATMENT. Open the victim's mouth, grasp the foreign object between your index and middle fingers, and try to remove the obstruction. If that doesn't work, place his head lower than his body or roll him on his side and slap his back.

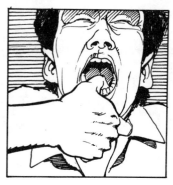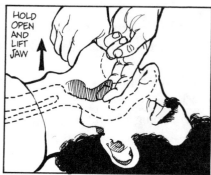

If the victim's breathing is impaired, open his mouth, lift his jaw, and remove the foreign object in his throat with two fingers.

If neither of these methods proves effective, try this:
1. Stand behind the choking victim with your arms around him just above the navel and below his rib cage.
2. Lean him forward at the waist with his head and arms hanging down.
3. Grasp your own wrist with your other hand and exert sudden very strong pressure against the victim's abdomen. This will force air out of his lungs and may expel the obstruction.

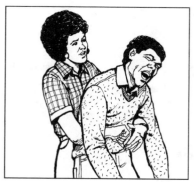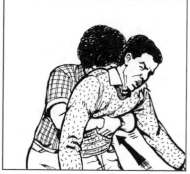

You stand behind the victim and exert pressure on his abdomen. This is commonly known as the "Heimlich manoeuvre."

Circulatory Failure

The causes of circulatory failure may be any one of four:
- Heart attack
- Impaired breathing
- Shock
- Electrical shock

The signs and symptoms are simply no breathing and no pulse.

FIRST-AID TREATMENT. *Do not waste time.* Cardiac arrest – that is, the heart has stopped beating – means certain death if cardiopulmonary resuscitation (CPR) is not attempted. But this treatment can only be performed by a person who has been properly trained to carry it out. If you have not been trained in CPR, then give mouth-to-mouth breathing and have someone call for emergency help urgently.

Severe Bleeding

Blood can come out of the body from one or more parts of the blood-carrying systems: arteries, veins, or capillaries. Depending on where the blood is coming from, there are distinct differences in the appearance of the blood and the way it flows.

These are signs and symptoms that will help you determine which system has been damaged and is bleeding:
- If an artery has been cut, the blood is bright red and spurts.
- If a vein has been severed, the blood is dark red and flows steadily.
- If the blood is coming from the capillary system, it oozes out.

FIRST-AID TREATMENT. 1. Cover the wound with the cleanest cloth immediately available or with your bare hand and apply direct pressure on the wound. Most bleeding can be stopped this way.

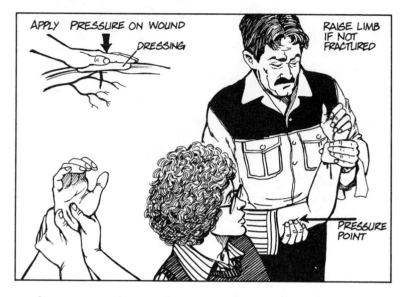

Apply pressure to the wound, raise the bleeding limb – if no bones are broken.

2. As you apply pressure, elevate the limb that has the cut – if there is no broken bone.
3. Use finger pressure at a pressure point if it is necessary to control bleeding from an arterial wound (bright red blood spurting from it). Apply your fingers to the appropriate pressure point – that is, the point where the main artery supplying blood to the wound is located. (See diagram on the following page.) Hold the pressure point tightly for about 5 *minutes* or until bleeding stops.

   The pressure points in the head and neck (there are three of them) should only be used as a *last resort* if there is a skull fracture and direct pressure cannot be used. If direct pressure can be used, it will stop bleeding on the head in about 95 per cent of injuries.
4. A tourniquet, a bandage tightened around a limb, should only be applied to an arm or leg *as a last resort*, if all other methods fail. A tourniquet is applied between the wound and the point at which the limb is attached to the body, as close to the wound as possible but never over the wound or

a fracture. Make sure it is applied tightly enough to stop bleeding completely. Once a tourniquet has been applied, care by a physician is imperative so as to prevent tissue deterioration and infection.

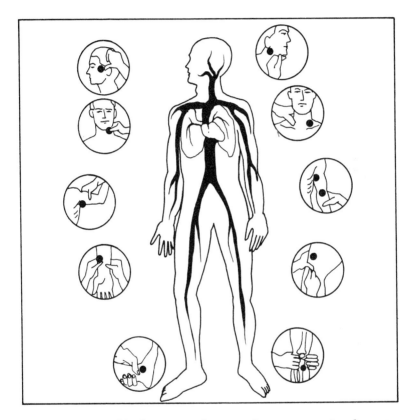

To control severe bleeding, press down on the pressure point closest to the wound – between the wound and the heart.

CAUTION

Once the serious decision has been made to use a tourniquet, it should *not* be loosened except on the advice of a physician, which must be sought immediately inasmuch as a tourniquet cannot be left on for more than a half-hour or so.

Internal bleeding, of course, offers no outward clues in the form of blood. But there are distinct signs and symptoms:
• Cold and clammy skin.
• A weak and rapid pulse.
• The eyes are dull and the pupils enlarged.
• Possible thirst.
• Nausea and vomiting.
• Pain in the affected area.

FIRST-AID TREATMENT. Treat the victim for shock immediately. Anticipate that he may vomit, so give him nothing by mouth even though he claims to be thirsty. Get the victim to medical assistance as quickly and as safely as possible.

Shock

Shock may accompany serious injury: blood loss, breathing impairment, heart failure, burns.

CAUTION

Shock can kill. Treat the patient as quickly as possible and continue treatment until medical aid is available.

There are distinctive signs and symptoms in patients suffering from shock:
• Shallow breathing
• Rapid and weak pulse
• Nausea, collapse, vomiting
• Shivering
• Pale, moist skin
• Mental confusion
• Drooping eyelids and dilated pupils

FIRST-AID TREATMENT. Make sure the patient can breathe easily. If necessary establish and maintain an open airway. If there is bleeding, get it under control immediately after you are sure that breathing is no problem. Finally, keep the patient lying down.

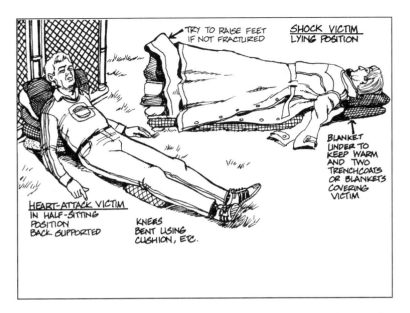

A semi-upright position is best for the victim of a heart attack or stroke (left). Keep shock victim (right) warm.

CAUTION

There are exceptions to keeping the shock patient lying down. If he has head and/or chest injuries, or has had a heart attack, stroke, or sun stroke, it is better to have the patient in a sitting position, or lying with the upper part of the body elevated.

If there has been no spine injury, the victim will be more comfortable and will breathe more easily if he is in a reclining position.

If you are in doubt, keep the victim lying down.

Unless his injury would be aggravated by elevating his feet, do so. Place blankets over – and under – him to help maintain his body temperature. Give him *nothing* by mouth – especially not stimulants or alcoholic beverages.

Remember, always treat for shock in all serious injuries and watch for it even in minor injuries.

Your First-Aid Primer

The following pages are devoted to the most common injuries or ailments for which you might have to give first aid. They are listed in alphabetical order to make it easier to find in an emergency and, where appropriate, are cross-referenced to other material in the book. Some techniques are also described where appropriate. The cross-referenced subjects are noted in the text in **bold** type.

Abdominal Injuries Wounds to the abdomen are particularly dangerous because there is a risk that internal organs have been damaged.

If the wound is deep, place the victim on his back with a pillow under the knees (to help relax the abdominal muscles). Get the bleeding under control and treat for **shock** (see page 150).

If the wound is open, *do not* try to replace **protruding intestines** or abdominal organs. Cover them with a sterile dressing, a clean towel, plastic film, or metal foil. Dampen the dressing if there is a delay in getting medical assistance; use sterile water or cool boiled water, if available. Hold the dressing in place with a firm bandage, but *do not* cause constriction by making the bandage too tight. If the victim has trouble breathing, keep his head and shoulders elevated with a pillow or a folded coat. Get help as quickly as possible.

CAUTION

Do not give fluids or solid food to victims of abdominal injuries as surgery will be necessary.

Artificial Respiration Even though there may be some doubt as to whether the victim's heart is beating, artificial respiration should be attempted. The mouth-to-mouth or mouth-to-nose technique is the most practical method and is considered superior to any manual technique. It also can be administered while in the water, in a small boat, underneath wreckage, or in other places where immediate resuscitation is required.

The manual method is not recommended except when mouth-to-mouth resuscitation cannot be performed for some reason, such as when massive facial injuries completely prevent the mouth-to-mouth or mouth-to-nose method. If the manual method is justified, it should be administered in this way:

1. Place the victim face up. Keep his airway open by raising his shoulders several inches, placing a folded coat or other padding under the shoulders, and allow his head to tip back.
2. Kneel at the top of the victim's head, grasp his wrists and cross them over his lower chest. Keep holding his wrists.
3. Rock forward until your arms are approximately vertical and allow the weight of your upper body to exert even downward pressure on the patient's arms and chest, forcing air out of his lungs.

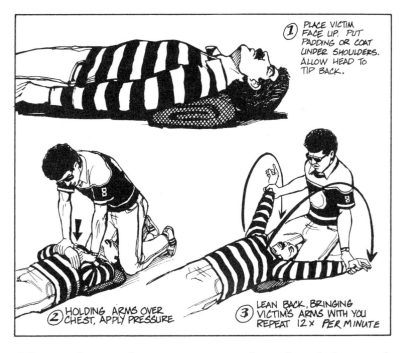

When mouth-to-mouth resuscitation cannot be performed, the manual method of resuscitation, though less desirable, may be used.

4. Rock back to release the pressure *immediately*, pulling the victim's arms outward and upward over his head, and backward as far as possible. This allows air to flow into his lungs.

5. Repeat about 12 times per minute.

6. Check the victim's mouth frequently for vomit or any other obstruction.

The mouth-to-mouth or mouth-to-nose method should be preceded by determining whether the victim is conscious. Tap him on the shoulder and inquire in a loud voice if he is all right.

1. Place the victim on his back. If it is necessary to roll him over, try to do it keeping his back and neck straight.

2. Kneel at his side, place one of your hands under his neck and the other on his forehead. Then tilt his head back so that his chin is pointing up.

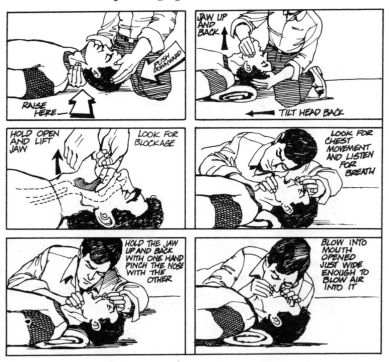

If the victim is conscious, mouth-to-mouth or mouth-to-nose resuscitation is commonly advised for artificial respiration.

3. Make sure his airway is not obstructed with food, tobacco, blood, dentures, etc. If there is an obvious obstruction, carefully turn the victim on his side, tilt his head down, and clear his mouth with your fingers. When the mouth is clear, return him to his back with head tilted as before.

4. Check for breathing by bending over the victim, and place your ear close to his mouth and nose. Listen for at least 5 seconds; feel for air exchange; look for chest movements.

5. If the victim is not breathing, pinch his nose closed with the hand you have resting on his forehead. Form an airtight seal by placing your mouth over his mouth, and breathe into his mouth until his chest rises. (If you are using the mouth-to-nose method, seal the victim's mouth with your hand and breathe in through his nose.)

6. Breathe into the victim 4 times as quickly as possible. If you do not feel or hear an air exchange, re-tilt his head and try again. If you still feel no air exchange, try clearing his mouth of any foreign objects and breathe into him again.

7. If there still is no air exchange, turn the victim on his side and slap him on the back between his shoulder blades. Again clear his mouth to remove any foreign matter. If none of the above steps clears the air passage, repeat the slaps on the back and tilt his head.

8. Repeat breathing. Remove mouth each time to allow air to escape. Repeat 12 times per minute for an adult, 20 times per minute for a small child or infant. As the victim begins to breathe, maintain head tilt.

CAUTION

While you would use deep breaths for an adult in mouth-to-mouth resuscitation, use smaller breaths for a child – and only gentle puffs for an infant.

Back Injuries Any accident that involves the back may have also involved the spine. Therefore, extremely careful handling of the victim is important. Do not bend his back during transportation.

If the victim requires **artificial respiration**, it should begin in the position in which he is lying.

A person who has been injured in the water should not have his head bent forward, nor should he be placed in a jackknife position. The victim should be floated to shore carefully and should be taken from the water only when rigid support is available.

Bandaging A bandage should be tight enough to prevent slipping, but not so tight as to cut off circulation.

CAUTION

Never tie a bandage around the neck. It could cause strangulation.

Leave fingers and toes exposed if uninjured, so that you can watch for swelling or changes of colour and so that you can feel for coldness – all of which signal interference with circulation.

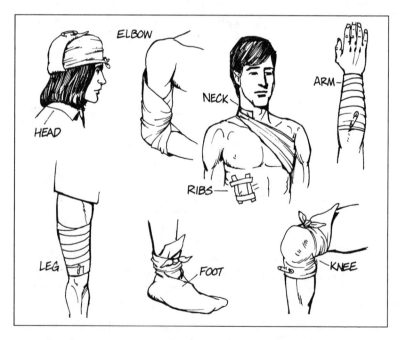

Some bandages may seem trickier to apply than others.

Loosen bandages immediately if the victim complains of numbness or a tingling sensation.

CAUTION

Once a dressing is in place, *do not* remove it. If blood saturates the dressing, put another on top of it.

Bites or Stings Animal bites should be washed with soap and water. Hold the wound under running water for two or three minutes if it is not bleeding profusely. Apply a sterile dressing and consult a physician. (See also **Open Wounds**.)

CAUTION

Protection against tetanus should be considered in treating a bite even if the skin appears intact.

Remember, the animal might have rabies. If you can do so safely, catch and cage it. Do *not* kill the animal because it may not be in an identifiable stage of the disease yet. Notify the police or the health department.

Insect stings cause serious allergic reactions in some people. Scrape out the stinger, if present, with a scraping motion of a fingernail. Do not pull it out. Avoid cold compresses. Consult a physician promptly if there is any reaction such as hives, generalized rash, pallor, weakness, nausea, vomiting, "tightness" in the chest, nose, or throat, or if the victim collapses.

Bites from non-poisonous snakes can be treated like cuts. Here again, tetanus protection should be considered. For treatment of bites from poisonous snakes, see **Snakebite**.

Bleeding The best way to control bleeding is with direct pressure over the site of the wound. Use a pad of sterile gauze, if one is available. Otherwise a clean handkerchief, sanitary napkin, or even the bare hand, if necessary, will do.

Apply firm, steady, direct pressure for 5 to 15 minutes. Most bleeding will stop within a few minutes.

If bleeding is from a hand, foot, arm, or leg, elevate the limb so that it is higher off the ground than the victim's heart. This will help to slow the flow.

Severe **nosebleed** can often be controlled by direct pressure, such as by pinching the nostrils with your fingers. Such pressure can be applied for up to 10 minutes without interruption.

Bleeding from the ear can indicate a **skull fracture**. If this is suspected, take care when trying to stop any scalp bleeding.

Remember, bleeding from the scalp can be very heavy even when the injury is superficial.

CAUTION

Don't press too hard when seeking to stop bleeding. Be especially careful when applying pressure over the wound, so that bone chips from a possible fracture will not be pressed into the brain.

Always suspect a neck injury when there is a serious head injury and immobilize the head and neck. Call for emergency help.

When the victim has suffered a head injury, *do not* give alcohol, cigarettes, or other drugs. They may mask important symptoms.

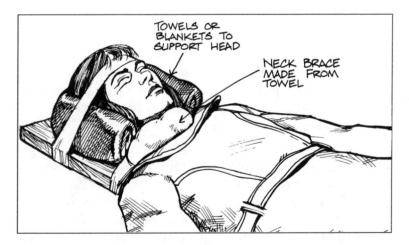

It's easy to keep the victim's head and neck immobile.

Should the victim cough up or vomit blood or material that looks like "coffee grounds," this could be a sign of internal bleeding. The victim might also pass blood in his urine or stool. His bowel movements may be black and tar-like. All of these symptoms indicate the need for immediate medical attention.

Have the victim lie flat and relax. Emergency help should be gotten immediately. *Do not* give any medication or fluids by mouth until a doctor has seen the victim and permits it.

Blisters Shoes or boots can cause blisters to appear on toes, heels, and the tops of feet. If *all* pressure can be relieved until the fluid is absorbed, it is best to leave the blister unbroken. Otherwise, wash the entire area with soap and water and make a small puncture at the base of the blister with a needle that has been sterilized by a match flame or by soaking in rubbing alcohol. Apply a sterile dressing and protect the area from further irritation.

If the blister has already broken, treat it as an **open wound**. Watch for signs of infection.

CAUTION

Do not attempt to care for a blister on your own hand or foot if it lies deep in the palm or on your sole.

Broken Bones Always remember that the victim *must not be moved* unless there is immediate danger of further injury. First check the victim's breathing. If needed, use **artificial respiration**. If there is bleeding, apply direct pressure over the site. If the victim is in **shock** (see page 150), keep him calm and warm. Call for emergency help.

CAUTION

Never try to push a broken bone into place if it is sticking out of the skin. Also, never try to straighten out a fracture.

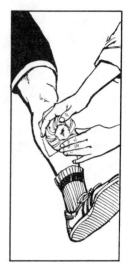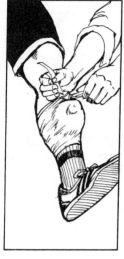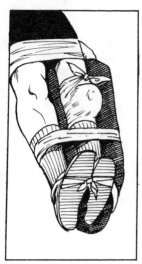

Immobilize the limb if an open fracture has occurred and the bone has pierced the skin. (See pages 173-174.)

If the broken bone is sticking out through the skin, apply a moist dressing to prevent drying out. Keep the victim immobile until emergency help arrives. If the fracture is unstable, try putting a simple splint around it to prevent painful motion.

Bruises Rest the injured part. Apply cold compresses for half an hour.

CAUTION

Never put ice next to the skin. Use an ice bag, or put the ice in a plastic bag and wrap the bag in a towel.

If the skin is broken, treat it as a **cut**. For washing-machine wringer injuries or bicycle-spoke injuries, consult a physician without delay.

Burns (chemical) Flood the affected area with clean water for at least 20 minutes until all traces of the chemical are removed. Then remove the victim's clothing lest any of the chemical is retained in the material.

CAUTION

Chemical burns of the eye require immediate medical attention after flushing with water for 20 minutes.

Burns (electric) If the burn has been caused by electricity, check immediately for **shock**. Do *not* use bare hands, but pull the victim away from the source of the current with non-conductive material. (See pages 124-126.)

Burns (heat) Reddened skin is the sign of a first-degree (surface) burn. Immerse in cold water or apply an ice bag or cold wet-packs to areas on the trunk or face to stop the burning process. Cooling must be constant until pain disappears. Non-adhesive dressings, or even plastic food-wrap, can be used as an emergency covering. Consult your physician.

If the skin is not only red but begins to blister, that is the sign of a second-degree burn. Cut away loose clothing from the affected area. Cover with several layers of cold, moist dressings, or if a limb is involved immerse in cold water for relief of pain. Treat for **shock** (see page 150.)

If the skin is destroyed, the tissues will be damaged and there will be visible charring. This is a third-degree burn. Cut away loose clothing – but *do not* try to remove clothing that has stuck to the skin. Cover the burned area with several layers of sterile, cold, moist dressings for relief of pain and to stop the burning action. Treat the victim for **shock** and call for help.

Burns (general care) If medical help is not available within an hour and the victim is conscious and not vomiting and he requests something to drink, mix a solution of 1/2 teaspoon salt and 1/2 teaspoon baking soda and one quart (one litre) of water. Allow the victim three ounces (1/2 glass) of the solution every 15 minutes.

When bandaging, separate any burned areas that might come in contact with each other, such as fingers, toes, ear and head. *Do not* use ointments, greases, powder, etc. Get medical attention as soon as possible.

CAUTION

Do not break blisters. Let them dry naturally.

Chest Wounds Cover the wound with an airtight material (aluminum foil or plastic wrap) after the victim has exhaled. If no airtight material is available, use your hand. Place the victim on his injured side to allow expansion room for the uninjured lung. Get the victim to a hospital as soon as possible.

Choking Anything stuck in the throat blocking the air passage can stop the breathing and cause unconsciousness and death within 4 to 6 minutes.

CAUTION

Do not interfere with a choking victim who can speak, cough, or breathe. However, if the choking continues without lessening, get emergency help.

If the victim cannot speak, cough, or breathe, have someone call for help while you give first aid.

If the patient is conscious, stand behind and to the side of him; he can be sitting or standing. Support him with one hand on his chest. Lower his head and apply 4 sharp blows between his shoulder blades. If this doesn't work, stand directly behind him, wrap your arms around him just above the navel and below the rib cage. Lean him forward at the waist with his head and arms hanging down, then grasp one of your wrists with the other hand and exert a strong upward thrust against his abdomen. Repeat this several times. If this still doesn't work, repeat the 4 back blows and give 4 upward thrusts. Continue this rotation of efforts until the victim is no longer choking – or becomes unconscious.

If the victim is unconscious, place him on the ground and give him **artificial respiration**. If the victim does not start

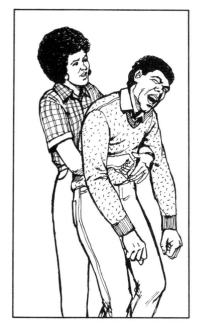 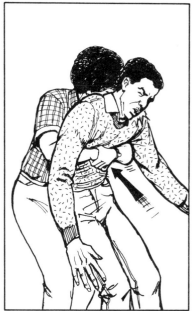

Use the Heimlich manoeuvre if the patient's air passage is blocked.

breathing and it appears that air is not entering his lungs, roll him onto his side, facing you, and place your knee against his chest. Give him 4 sharp blows between the shoulder blades. Should this still bring no response, roll him on his back.

Now place one of your hands on top of the other, with the heel of the bottom hand in the middle of his abdomen slightly above the navel and below the rib cage. Press his abdomen with a quick upward thrust – but *do not* press to either side. Repeat 4 times if needed. Clear his airway by following the instructions given on pages 145-146.

Remember, keep repeating these treatments – in a rotation: 4 back blows, 4 abdominal thrusts, clear the airway, try to inflate his lungs . . . and repeat until successful.

Choking (child) If the child chokes and is not breathing, turn him over your knees, head and face down, and forcefully hit his back between the shoulder blades in an effort to dislodge the object from his windpipe. If he can breathe, do not attempt this manoeuvre.

CAUTION

If an object blocking the throat has not been retrieved – whether the victim is child or adult – but the swallower suddenly seems all right, play it safe: take him to the hospital. This is especially critical if the object swallowed is a fish bone, chicken bone, or other jagged object that can cause internal damage.

Closed Wounds A closed wound can occur anywhere within the body. No skin break will occur, and no blood will be lost through the skin, though it may flow through outer openings of body cavities. Closed wounds are less likely to become infected than **open wounds**, since they are subject to less contamination. Many closed wounds are relatively small injuries involving soft tissue – such as a black eye. Others, however, may involve extensive internal bleeding as well as severe physical damage to tissue, organs, or systems.

Most closed wounds are caused by external forces – falls, car accidents, etc. However, a closed wound can be caused if the victim of a closed fracture is mishandled or is moved before a splint is properly applied to immobilize the injury.

Even if no outward signs of injury are obvious, internal injury is possible when any one of the following symptoms is present:
• Cold, clammy, pale skin.
• Very rapid but weak pulse.
• Rapid breathing and dizziness.
• Pain and tenderness in a part of the body in which the injury is suspected, especially if a deep pain continues and seems disproportionate to the injury symptoms.
• Excessive thirst.
• Uncontrolled restlessness.
• Vomited or coughed-up blood.
• Blood in the urine or feces.

Pain and tenderness will be accompanied by swelling, discolouration, and possibly deformity of limbs caused by **fractures** or **dislocations**.

Take the following actions:
- Make sure the airway is open; give **artificial respiration** if needed.
- Examine for fractures and injuries to head, neck, chest, abdomen, limbs, back, and spine.
- Get medical help immediately if you suspect internal injury.
- If a closed **fracture** is suspected, immobilize the affected area before moving the victim.
- If he must be moved, make sure he is lying down while being transported – and be careful not to cause shock.

CAUTION

Do not give the victim anything to drink if there is internal injury or the suspicion of it – no matter how much he complains of thirst.

If the closed wound is relatively small (like a black eye), put cold applications on the injured area to prevent added tissue swelling and to slow down internal bleeding. Warm applications should never be used; they encourage bleeding.

Convulsions A convulsion is an attack of unconsciousness that usually comes on violently. In infants and small children, convulsions can develop due to an acute infectious disease. As the child becomes older, convulsions can develop during some of the childhood diseases like measles or mumps, and this situation is considered serious. Convulsions are also associated with head injuries or disease.

The child's muscles become rigid for a period of a few seconds up to a half-minute. This body rigidity is followed by jerky movements. During the period of rigidity, the child may stop breathing, bite his tongue severely, and lose control of bladder and bowels. The face and lips will turn blue, and the child will drool or foam at the mouth before the symptoms subside.

The first thing you must do is prevent the child from hurting himself. Lay the child on his side with his head lower than the hips. Apply cold cloths to his head and sponge him with cool water. If it seems necessary, give him **artificial respiration**.

CAUTION

Do not place anything in a child's mouth if he is having a convulsion – no liquids, and especially nothing placed between his teeth to prevent him from biting his tongue. Do not place him in a tub of water.

If repeated convulsions occur, call for medical assistance or take the child to a hospital immediately. In any case, if your child has had a convulsion, consult a physician.

Cuts If the cut is small, wash it with soap and water. Hold the cut under running water for a while, then apply a sterile dressing. If the cut is large, clean and rinse it, then apply a dressing. Press firmly and elevate the part of the body that has the cut to help stop the bleeding. Bandage and get medical attention. If the victim is a child and the cut is large, *do not* use iodine or other antiseptics before a physician has seen the patient.

Diabetic Emergencies If a sufferer of diabetes suddenly begins deep rapid breathing, this may be a sign of a diabetic coma. The victim's temperature will drop, his skin will be red and dry, and there will be a sickly sweet odour of acetone on his breath. Treat the victim as you would for **shock** (see page 150). Place him in a semi-reclining position. If he should vomit, turn his head to one side. *Do not* give him any sugar, carbohydrates, fats, or alcoholic beverages.

A diabetic can sometimes suffer from insulin shock. His skin will be pale, moist, and clammy and he will be covered in a cold sweat. His breathing will be normal or shallow, and there will be no odour of acetone (like nail-polish remover) on his breath.

This is a critical emergency: first-aid treatment should be given quickly:
- If the victim is conscious, give him sugar (candy bar, orange juice, sugar); or
- If the victim is unconscious, put sugar *under* the tongue.

Because it is difficult to determine the difference between the diabetic emergencies, sugar should be given to any unconscious or semi-conscious diabetic, even though he may be suffering from diabetic coma (too much sugar). The reason for doing this is that an insulin reaction (too little sugar) resulting in unconsciousness can quickly cause brain damage or death.

Dislocations These can occur as a result of a fall or a direct blow. Unless given proper care, such displacement of a bone-end from a joint – particularly at the shoulder, elbow, fingers, or thumb – may occur repeatedly.

Swelling, discolouration, and obvious deformity are the immediate outward signs of the problem. The victim will experience pain when trying to move the joint as well as tenderness to the touch. Immobilize the affected joint – using a splint if necessary – in the position it is. Use a sling, if appropriate. If a limb is involved, elevate the affected part. Get medical attention promptly.

CAUTION

Do not try to replace a dislocated bone-end into its joint.

Just as you have been cautioned not to attempt readjusting the dislocation, so should you be cautioned not to try to reduce the swelling or correct any deformity near the joint. Careless handling of the victim may cause serious internal damage at the area of the dislocation.

See also **Fracture (closed)** and **Spine Fracture**.

Drowning Victims of drowning can die within 4 to 6 minutes of the accident because they have stopped breathing.

Therefore, it is essential that you get the victim out of the water at once. It is best to avoid direct contact with him, if possible, since a panicked victim may drown the rescuer as well. If he is conscious, push a floating object to him or let him grasp a long branch, pole, or other similar object. If he is unconscious, take a flotation device with you if possible and approach the victim with caution. Once ashore, or on the deck of a boat or pool, he should be placed on his back.

If he is not breathing, start **artificial respiration** immediately. Continue until the victim can breathe unassisted. That can take an hour or two, so pace yourself – keep calm.

Remember, even when the victim is breathing unassisted, he may be in need of medical attention. Have someone else go for help. Do not leave the victim alone under any circumstances, not even to call for help.

If the victim is breathing without assistance – even though coughing and sputtering – he will get rid of the water remaining in his system. You need only stand by to see that recovery continues. Send someone else for assistance.

Drug Overdose You must think of such an occurrence as a poisoning. Alcohol is as much a poison as stimulants, tranquilizers, narcotics, hallucinogens, or inhalants. Don't take drunkenness lightly – too much alcohol can kill.

Get emergency help at once. Check the victim's breathing and pulse. If his breathing has stopped, or is very weak, give **artificial respiration**.

CAUTION

A victim being revived from alcohol poisoning can be violent. Be careful.

Until help arrives, make sure he is still breathing. Cover him with a blanket. Do not throw water in his face – and *do not* give liquor or a stimulant: alcohol in combination with certain drugs can be deadly.

Electric Shock Normal electric current can be deadly (see Chapter Two). Do not touch a person who has been in contact with electric current until you are certain that the electricity has been turned off. It is best to turn if off at the main switch. If that is impossible or difficult, pull the plug out of the socket.

If the victim is in contact with a wire or a downed power line, use a dry stick or other non-conductor to move the line away. (See pages 124-126.)

Check for breathing. If the victim's breathing is weak or has stopped, give **artificial respiration** immediately. Send for emergency help, keep the victim warm (cover him with a coat, blanket, etc.), but *do not* give him anything to drink or eat until a physician has seen him.

Epileptic Seizure The victim may lose consciousness, have convulsions or severe spasm of the muscles of the jaw (he may bite his tongue), or vomit. His face will become red and the veins in his neck will be swollen. Breathing may be loud and laboured with a hissing sound. A seizure may only last a few minutes, but it could be followed by another.

It is important that *you* keep calm.

Don't restrain the victim. Instead, move away any objects that could be dangerous to him. Place light padding under his head (coat, jacket, shirt, rug).

There is a danger of the victim biting his tongue, so place a padded object between his jaws on one side of his mouth – a rolled handkerchief or shirt tail on a stick, for example. *Do not* try to force his jaws open if they are already clamped shut.

When the seizure is over, loosen clothing around his neck. Keep him lying down and see that his airway is open. Turn his head sideways – or turn him on his stomach – to prevent him from breathing vomit into his lungs. If he stops breathing, give **artificial respiration**.

When the seizure is over and the victim is conscious, allow him to sleep or rest.

Eye Injuries To remove a foreign body from the eye, try to flush it out with clean water, or use a moist cotton swab – but don't overdo it. For chemical burns to the eyes, flushing with clean water is especially important – see **Burns (chemical)**.

CAUTION

Don't allow the eye-injury victim to rub his eyes.

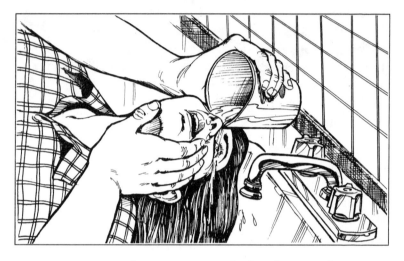

Treat eye injuries with care to prevent further damage. This victim's eye is being flushed with water after a chemical burn.

If the foreign object is under the upper lid, lift the eyelid and remove the object with sterile gauze.

If the foreign object is on the eye and cannot be washed out, place sterile gauze around the eye, but apply no pressure. Cover with a paper cup or cardboard cone, to protect it and prevent the object from being driven further into the eye. It is advisable then to cover both eyes, since one eye cannot move without the other eye moving. Take the victim to a physician. Pain in the eye from foreign bodies or scrapes, scratches, and cuts can be reduced by bandaging the lid shut until medical aid can be obtained.

CAUTION

Never use drops or ointment in an eye-injury emergency.

Fainting Fainting is a partial or complete loss of consciousness due to reduced supply of blood to the brain for a short time. Recovery of consciousness almost always occurs when the victim is placed in a flat position – or falls.

To prevent a fainting attack, a person who feels weak and dizzy should lie down or bend over with his head at the level of his knees.

If the victim has fainted, leave him in a flat position. Loosen clothing around the neck and then any other tight clothing. Should he vomit, roll him on his side or turn his head to one side. Wipe out his mouth if necessary, using your fingers (preferably wrapped in cloth). Make sure his airway remains open.

CAUTION

Do not splash water on the face of someone who has fainted or give him anything to drink – unless he is *fully* conscious.

If the victim fell, check for injury. Keep him warm. Unless recovery is prompt, seek medical assistance.

Foot Injuries (See **Leg Injuries**)

Fracture (closed) This is known as a simple fracture. That is, there is a broken bone but no open wound. If the victim is conscious, he will usually be able to provide clues to possible fractures. He may recall his position before the injury and relate what happened as he fell or struck some object. In addition, he may have heard or felt a bone snap. He might be able to indicate the location of pain and tenderness and may have some difficulty in moving the injured part. He may have a sensation of broken bones rubbing together.

Outwardly you might see some deformity in the area of the break as well as discolouration, swelling – and, if it is an open fracture, exposed bone. See **Fracture (open)**.

Closed fractures are much more common than open fractures. As a rule, diagnosis can be made only by a physician with the assistance of an X-ray examination. If there is any doubt that the victim has suffered a fracture, proceed with first-aid treatment.

Dislocations are similar to closed fractures. A **dislocation** occurs when two bones that come together to form a joint are separated. Here again you likely will see some deformity. The victim will report pain and will suffer a loss of the function of the joint.

If you suspect a fracture, keep the victim quiet and still. Make sure the airway is open and apply **artificial respiration**, if indicated. Call for medical assistance. If you can do it without disturbing the suspected fracture, elevate the extremity involved. If medical help is not immediately available, you may have to try to apply a splint. The victim should not be moved and should be handled as gently as possible. Splinting should be done in pairs, one person to immobilize the limb and one to apply the splint.

If you must make a splint, an umbrella, a board, or any other stiff object may be used. Cover it with something soft, such as clothing or bed linen. Make sure the splint extends beyond joints, to restrict motion. With a fractured limb, a useful splint is a folded pillow that is loosely tied to the arm or leg.

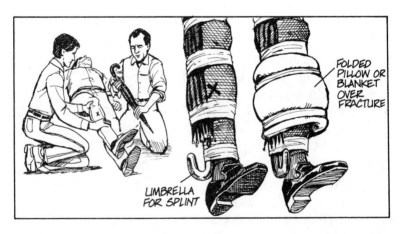

FOLDED PILLOW OR BLANKET OVER FRACTURE

UMBRELLA FOR SPLINT

If you must improvise a splint, use your ingenuity to make one that will work effectively to hold an injured limb immobile.

If the victim has suffered a fracture, place the part of the body affected in as nearly normal a position as possible by applying slight traction. Traction is applied by grasping the affected limb gently but firmly, with one hand above and the other below the location of the fracture, and pulling the limb between your hands. This is maintained until the second person can secure the splint in place.

CAUTION

Never try to straighten the bone if a joint or the spine is involved.

In the case of a **dislocation**, immobilize the joint in the position it was when you came to the victim's aid. *Do not* attempt to reduce or straighten any dislocation.

Fracture (open) In an open fracture, a wound is usually caused by a broken bone-end that tears through the skin and, in most cases, slips back again. Open fractures are much more serious because of tissue damage and bleeding and danger of infection – the fracture area is always contaminated.

Do not attempt to set (or reduce) a fracture or try to push a protruding bone-end back. If transportation is necessary, the bone-end may slip back when the limb is straightened for splinting. If emergency transportation is not immediately available, *do not* attempt to move the victim unless there is danger of fire, carbon monoxide poisoning, explosion, drowning, or other life-threatening emergency.

Remember, if you have to rescue a victim, do not drag him out of a vehicle or from under wreckage or throw him on the ground in haste to save his life. If possible, even in the middle of a crowded street or highway, take the time to tie the victim's injured leg to his uninjured one, or bind his injured arm to his chest or side, so that the injured limb is immobilized.

If the victim is unconscious, lift and move him as though he has an injury to his neck or spine. Wait for adequate help – at least three other persons – so that, if possible, you can get rigid support for his back as you lift him.

If the victim has suffered a neck or spinal injury during water activity, float him to shore without bending his neck or back. *Do not* lift him out of the water without back support.

If an open fracture is evident or suspected, treat the wound (see **Open Wounds**), then remove or cut away the victim's clothes in the area of the damage. To control hemorrhage, apply pressure with a large sterile (or clean) dressing placed over the wound. If a fragment of bone is protruding, cover the entire wound with a large, sterile bandage, compress, or pads. If these are not available, use freshly laundered towels or sheets.

• **Do not** wash the wound.
• **Do not** probe the wound.
• **Do not** insert your fingers into the wound.
• **Do not** replace bone fragments.

If you have applied a splint, elevate the limb to reduce hemorrhage and swelling.

Frostbite The most frequently frostbitten parts of the body are toes, fingers, nose, and ears that have been exposed to cold. The skin becomes pale or greyish yellow. The patient will say that the affected parts feel cold and numb, and they will feel doughy to the touch.

Until the victim can be brought inside, he should be wrapped in woollen cloth and kept dry. *Do not* rub, chafe, or manipulate frostbitten parts. When you have brought the victim indoors, place him in warm water (102°F to 105°F; 39°C to 41°C) and make sure it remains warm. Test the water temperature by pouring it on the inner surface of your forearm. Never thaw the victim if he has to go back into the cold; this may cause the affected area to be refrozen.

Do not use hot water bottles or a heat lamp, and don't place the victim near a hot stove. If his feet are affected, *do not* allow him to walk.

Once he has thawed, have the victim gently exercise the affected parts. If the frostbite is serious, seek medical aid for thawing, because the pain will be intense and tissue damage can be extensive.

Genital Injuries Injuries to the genital organs may result from kicks, blows, straddle accidents, accidents involving machinery, and even blows from sharp instruments. There is great pain and the organs can swell markedly and even bleed profusely.

Remember, save any torn tissue for possible skin grafting. (See **Open Wounds**.)

Bleeding should be controlled by direct pressure with the hand on a cloth pad. If necessary, treat for *shock*. Use protective and supportive dressings for any wounds that are open, and apply cold packs. Rest is necessary.

Hand Injuries Elevate the injured hand above the level of the heart. This will reduce swelling. (Only after **snakebite** and other **bites or stings** should the hand be allowed to hang down.) If the wound is quite serious, *do not* try to cleanse it.

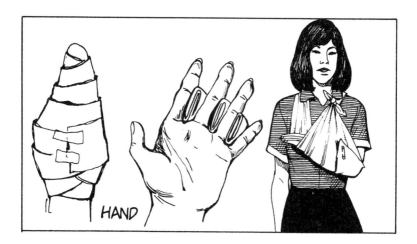

Separate the fingers with pads of gauze before bandaging an injured hand.

Place a sterile pad over the wound to control bleeding, then apply pressure by placing a roll of bandage or other material in the palm of the victim's hand and have him curve his fingers around it. Separate the fingers with gauze pads and cover the hand with a clean cloth or a plastic bag that has never been used. Place the arm in a sling with the hand as high as it can go and transport the victim for emergency treatment. (See also **Open Wounds**.)

Handling Casualties Unless the victim is in serious danger of death by remaining where he is, always try to stop bleeding before trying to move him. Keep the victim warm to reduce shock. If the accident occurred in such a way that he is lying among debris, clear dust and dirt from his mouth and nose and protect him from any further falling debris. If necessary, give **artificial respiration**. Cut free any clothing that has been caught by debris or by anything else.

CAUTION

When treating a patient who is lying amid debris, do not move debris – you could cause a further collapse of the damaged structure.

If you must move the victim quickly and you are alone, there are several methods you can use:

FIREMAN'S CRAWL. Use a triangular bandage, a torn shirt, etc., to tie the victim's hands together at the wrists. Place him flat on his back; then place yourself over him, on hands and knees, with your head between his tied-together arms, placing his wrists on your neck. Then crawl forward, straddling his body as you drag him.

HUMAN CRUTCH. If the victim is only slightly hurt and can help himself, place one of his arms over your shoulder, putting your hand behind his back and around his waist. He can then walk with your support.

PIGGY-BACK. If he is conscious but too weak to walk with you as a human crutch, lift him onto your back as you would to carry a child piggy-back. Do not try this if the victim is not conscious.

MOVING DOWN A FLIGHT OF STAIRS. Again, tie the hands at the wrists with a triangular bandage or some other large piece of cloth. With the victim on his back, place his tied-together wrists behind your head and walk down the stairs backward, supporting his shoulders with your hands so that he does not bang his head on the steps as you drag him backward with you. *Do not* do this if the victim has broken limbs.

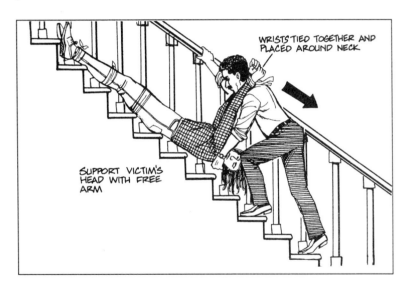

Moving a patient down a flight of stairs is easier this way.

If you must move the victim quickly and *there are two of you,* here are several useful methods:

FORE-AND-AFT METHOD. Place your arms under the victim's armpits and join your hands around his chest; the other person places his hands under the victim's knees. Then lift and carry. This is a useful way to carry an injured person if the injury is not serious, and it can be used if he is unconscious.

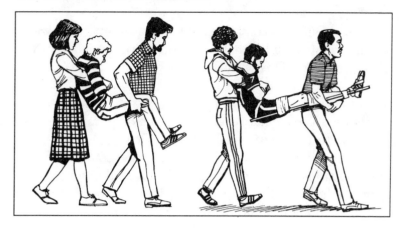

Modify the usual fore-and-aft carry (left) if the patient's leg is broken (right). (See cautionary note below.)

CAUTION

If the victim has a broken leg, you must tie the legs together so that the uninjured leg acts as a splint; then carry both legs over one arm.

TWO-HANDED SEAT CARRY. Stand on either side of the victim. Make a seat by hooking together the fingers on your "outside" arms (the person on the left uses his left arm; the person on the right uses his right arm) to make a swing-type seat; and use the two "inside" arms as a backrest. Always pad your hooked-together fingers with a handkerchief to prevent damaging each other's hand with your nails.

FOUR-HANDED SEAT CARRY. An ideal way to carry a conscious victim. Each carrier grasps his right wrist with his left hand. Then each grasps the other's left wrist and his own right hand. The victim, sitting on the four-handed seat, puts his arms around the shoulders of the carriers.

CHAIR LIFT. If you have a straight-back chair that is strong enough to bear the weight of the victim, sit him upright. One carrier grasps the front legs of the chair, the other the back of the chair. Tilt the chair backward to a 45° angle and carry forward much as with a stretcher.

Head Injuries Special attention must be taken when trying to stop any bleeding from the scalp if there is a suspected skull fracture. Bleeding from the scalp can be very heavy even when the injury is not too serious.

CAUTION

If there is bleeding from an ear, it can mean there is a skull fracture.

When applying a sterile pad to the source of the bleeding, don't press too hard because any undue pressure could force bone chips from a skull fracture into the brain.

Remember, always suspect a neck injury when there is a serious head injury. Immobilize both head and neck.

Get medical help immediately. And while awaiting emergency services *do not* give the victim alcohol, cigarettes, or other drugs. They could mask important symptoms.

Head Injuries to Children Insist on complete rest and consult a physician immediately if:
• There is loss of consciousness at the time of the injury or any time thereafter.
• You are unable to rouse the child from sleep. You may allow the child to sleep after the injury, but check frequently to see whether he can be aroused. Check at least every 1 or 2 hours during the day, and 2 or 3 times during the night.
• There is persistent vomiting. Many children vomit immediately from fright, but vomiting should not persist.
• There is an inability to move a limb.
• There is blood or watery fluid oozing from the child's ears or nose.
• The child complains of a persistent headache for more than one hour. The headache will be severe enough to interfere with activity and normal sleep.

- There is persistent dizziness for one hour after the injury.
- The child's pupils are not equal in size. Be sure that a light is not shining in one eye which could cause that pupil to become smaller.
- The child's complexion is pallid and does not return to normal in a short time.

Heart Attack While this is the number-one killer of adults over the age of 38, many heart attack victims die needlessly because they did not get help in time. Warning signs include shortness of breath; crushing pain in the chest under the breastbone, or pain radiating through either the left arm, the neck, or the jaw; sweating and weakness; nausea or vomiting; pain that extends across the shoulders to the back; ashen colour and anxiety.

CAUTION

If the victim is experiencing any of the sensations described above, take no chances – call for emergency help at once. Victims most often deny they are having a heart attack and try to reject assistance.

Two critical life-threatening things happen to the victim of a heart attack:
- Breathing slows down or stops.
- The heart may slow down or stop pumping blood.

Place the victim in a semi-reclining or sitting position. Loosen tight clothing at the neck and waist. If oxygen is available, administer it. Ask the victim if he is carrying nitroglycerine pills; if so, place one under his tongue. If the pain is not relieved in a minute or so, you may administer a second pill.

Comfort the victim and reassure him. *Do not* allow him to move around – and *do not* give him any stimulants. Keep onlookers away.

If the victim is not breathing, have someone call for emergency help while you administer **artificial respiration**.

Heat Cramp People who are working or doing strenuous exercise in a hot environment are susceptible to heat cramp. The muscles of the legs and abdomen are likely to be affected first, and the cramps can be very painful. The victim will feel faint and will perspire profusely. If you must do hard work in high temperatures, drink large amounts of cool water with a pinch of salt added to each glassful.

Move the victim to a cool place. Exert firm pressure with your hands on the cramped muscles, or gently massage them, to help relieve the spasm. Give the victim sips of salted drinking water (using one teaspoon of salt to a quart or litre of water), over a period of about one hour.

Heat Exhaustion The victim will turn pale, his skin will become clammy, and he will perspire profusely. His breathing will be rapid and shallow. He will feel weak, dizzy, and develop a headache.

Treat the victim as though he is in **shock** (see page 150). Move him to a cool area, but *do not* allow him to become chilled. If his body gets too cold, cover him.

Heat Stroke The victim's face will become red and flushed, his skin hot and dry, with no perspiration. He will rapidly become unconscious.

Lay the victim down with head and shoulders raised. Reduce the body temperature as quickly as possible by administering cold applications to his head and body and using a fan if available. Get medical help as quickly as possible.

Hypothermia This is the primary killer of winter sports enthusiasts: subnormal body temperature. It is discussed fully in Chapter Nine.

Insect Bites (See **Bites or Stings**)

Internal Bleeding (See **Bleeding**)

Leg Injuries Serious wounds to the legs and feet are obviously incapacitating, but they can be life-threatening and this fact is often overlooked. Persons with poor circulation – particularly older people — find that such injuries take longer to heal.

Injuries to legs and feet should receive medical attention. But if this cannot be given immediately, cover the wound and wrap it with supportive, but not constrictive, bandages. Keep the injured limb elevated on a pillow or a rolled-up coat or blanket. *Do not* allow the victim to walk. If possible, keep the victim from putting his shoes and stockings back on. If this cannot be done, then remove the victim's shoes and stockings from time to time to examine the toes. If they become swollen and blue, loosen the bandages but *do not* remove the dressings.

Neck Injuries The victim's airway can become blocked due to an excessive flow of body fluids from damaged tissue in the throat area. Swelling can also occur and block the airway. If necessary, use **artificial respiration**. Should the airway need to be opened surgically, get medical help immediately.

Cuts or puncture wounds of the neck may involve the jugular veins (on both sides of the neck just beneath the surface of the skin), or major arteries and veins deeper in the flesh. Bleeding from neck wounds is dangerous and difficult to control. This is the method to use to attempt bleeding control:
1. Make sure the victim's airway is open.
2. Exert direct pressure over the wound with a gauze pad.
3. Keep the victim's head and shoulders raised.
4. Seek medical assistance without delay.

If bleeding is not a problem, cover the wound with a dressing held in place with tape.

CAUTION

Never apply a circular bandage around the neck.

Nosebleed Place the victim in a sitting position and have him blow out all the clot and blood. Into the bleeding nostril insert a wedge of cotton that has been moistened with any of the common nose drops. If nose drops are not available, moisten the cotton with hydrogen peroxide or cold water. Apply firm pressure with your fingers against the outside of the bleeding nostril for 5 minutes. If the bleeding persists, seek medical assistance.

Open Fractures (See **Fracture**)

Open Wounds An open wound is a break in the skin or the mucous membrane. There are five types:

ABRASIONS. Skin is scraped off the flesh; bleeding is limited; there is a danger of contamination and infection.

AVULSIONS. Tissue or skin is forcibly separated or torn loose from the body, or is left hanging as a flap. Body parts that have been partly or wholly torn off (such as ear lobes, fingers – even entire limbs) may sometimes successfully be reattached by a surgeon. In such a case, collect the separated part or parts and place them in a clean plastic bag. Then place the sealed bag in iced water and take it along with the patient to the medical facility. Do not immerse the part in water directly. Note: If a tooth is knocked out of the jaw, it may be replaceable similarly and should be saved in the same way and taken to the dentist or medical facility.

INCISIONS. Skin is cut by a sharp object; bleeding may be heavy and rapid; muscles, tendons, and nerves could be damaged.

LACERATIONS. Skin or tissue is torn open; bleeding may be extensive and rapid; deep contamination could lead to serious infection.

PUNCTURE. Skin is pierced; external bleeding is usually limited; internal damage to organs is possible with resulting heavy internal bleeding; hazards of infection are great and tetanus may develop.

First stop the bleeding and cover with a sterile dressing (or the cleanest cloth available at the moment). If the wound involves a surface area with little bleeding, wash with soap and water.

CAUTION

If an object is imbedded in the flesh, *do not* remove it. Instead, cut away clothing from the injury site; stabilize the object with bulky dressings; cover the object with a paper cup or cardboard cone, if possible, or apply a bandage to prevent any movement of the object. Get medical assistance.

If you have to transport a patient with an object impaled in his flesh, and the object is too large to allow for transportation, cut off enough to permit his being moved.

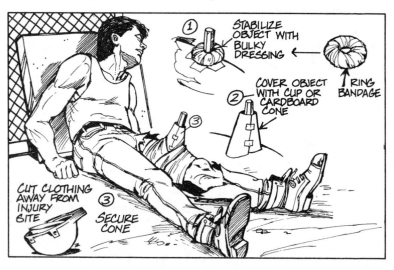

Do not remove an object imbedded in a victim. Protect the injury until medical help is available.

Poison The average home is loaded with poisons and children are most vulnerable. Call a physician, poison control centre, or the nearest hospital emergency room immediately. If the patient is conscious and not convulsing, dilute the poison by having him drink a glass of water or milk. If he becomes nauseated, stop the dilution process. You might induce vomiting by administering syrup of ipecac (for children: one tablespoon or one-half ounce, followed by a cup of water; for adults: two tablespoons or one ounce). If no vomiting occurs in 20 minutes, you may repeat the dose *once* only.

CAUTION

Do not induce vomiting if a victim has swallowed kerosene or other petroleum products, furniture polish, paint thinner, or a strong corrosive such as lye or acids, or if the victim is convulsing or unconscious.

If syrup of ipecac is not available, vomiting may be induced by tickling the back of the victim's throat with a finger or the *blunt* end of a spoon, fork, or knife.

Save the label or container of the suspected poison for identification. If the victim vomits, save a sample for analysis.

If the victim becomes unconscious, keep his airway open. Use **artificial respiration** and call for emergency help at once. *Do not* give liquids to an unconscious person or induce vomiting. If the victim is vomiting of his own accord, position him and turn his head so that the vomit drains out of his mouth.

If the victim is having convulsions, call for emergency assistance immediately. *Do not* attempt to restrain him, but position him in such a way that he will not injure himself. Loosen tight clothing at the victim's neck and waist. If he is having trouble breathing, use **artificial respiration**. Do not give liquids or force anything between his teeth. *Do not* induce vomiting.

Protruding Intestines If the abdomen has been punctured or torn and the intestines are exposed, *do not* attempt to replace them. Leave the exposed organ on the surface and cover it with non-adherent material such as aluminum foil or plastic wrap. Then cover with an outer dressing to hold everything in place while awaiting emergency services.

Rib Fractures The first symptom of a rib fracture is pain, localized at the site of the fracture. By asking the victim to place his hand on the exact area of the pain, if he is conscious, you can determine the location of the injury. Other signs of a rib fracture are rib deformity or lacerations, or a tendency on the part of the victim to lean toward the injured side with his hand held over the injury site in an attempt to ease the pain and immobilize the chest. The victim will say that deep breathing, coughing, or any movement is painful.

Place the arm on the injured side across the victim's chest with the elbow at the waist and the hand pointing up toward the opposite shoulder. Now bind the arm to the chest using two long bandages or neckties. With a third bandage, make a support for the arm that is angled toward the shoulder. The bandages should be tightened while the victim has exhaled.

CAUTION

In immobilizing an arm to ease a rib injury, make certain the binding is not too tight, as a fractured rib might puncture a lung.

Scrapes Use gauze or cotton to gently sponge off the scraped area with soap and water. Apply a sterile dressing, preferably of the non-adhesive or "film" type. If the skin is broken, consider the possibility of protection against tetanus.

Seizure It's alarming to see the victim – limbs jerking violently, eyes rolling upward, and breathing becoming heavy with dribble or froth at the lips. In some seizures, breathing may stop or the victim may bite his tongue so severely that it bleeds and obstructs the airway. However, you must *not* try to force anything into the victim's mouth to prevent tongue-biting.

There is little you can do to stop the seizure, so allow it to run its course, but call for help. When the attack is over, help the victim lie down to keep him from falling. Loosen restrictive clothing.

CAUTION

Never try to restrain a seizure victim. Do not use force on him. Move objects out of the way if they could injure him as his limbs jerk around. If an object that might cause him harm cannot be moved, put clothing or soft material between him and the object.

After the seizure check to see if he is breathing. If he is not, give **artificial respiration**.

Remember, if there are any burns around the mouth, the seizure could have been caused by poison. Follow procedures for **poison** treatment.

The victim may be conscious but confused and not talkative when the intense movement stops. Stay with him. Be certain breathing continues. Then seek medical assistance when he seems able to move.

Skull Fracture If you suspect a skull fracture, look for these signs and symptoms: deformity of the skull, an open wound, blood or water-like fluid coming from the ears or nose, and the victim's pupils unequal in size (provided a bright light is not shining into one of his eyes). He might, of course, also be unconscious.

First, make sure the airway is open. Check for spinal injury and keep the victim quiet.

If there is no suspected neck or spine injury, turn the head so that it does not rest on the fracture. Place the victim on his back and raise his head and shoulders, or place him in a three-quarter prone position. Use an ice pack to stop severe bleeding.

CAUTION

Do not stop bleeding from ears and nose if you suspect a skull fracture. Get medical assistance quickly.

Slivers Wash the affected part with soap and water. Then remove the splinter with a pair of tweezers or forceps. Then wash the area again. If the sliver is large or deep, seek medical help.

Snakebite Puncture marks are the first physical sign of a snake's bite. The victim of a bite from a poisonous snake likely will experience nausea and vomiting as well as respiratory distress. He may complain of severe burning and pain at the location of the bite and there may be a spreading swelling. Watch for **shock** (see page 150).

Immobilize the victim immediately, with the injured part lower than the rest of the body. Keep him quiet: any activity will stimulate the spread of the poison. Remove rings, watches, and/or bracelets. Apply a constricting band above the swelling caused by the bite. It should be tight, but not tight enough to stop arterial circulation.

Make an incision, no more than 1/8 inch (3 mm) deep, and no more than about half-inch (1 cm) lengthwise through the fang marks. Press around the cut to make it bleed. Suction the wound with your mouth (if you have no open sores in your mouth or on your lips) and spit out the blood.

Remember, cutting and suction is of no value unless done immediately.

CAUTION

Do not cut into a snakebite victim's flesh if the bite is near a major artery.

If the swelling continues past the constricting band, put on another band beyond the swelling and loosen the first band.

Treat the victim for **shock** and do not give him any stimulants or alcohol. Identify the snake if possible. If it can be killed, take it to the hospital with the victim.

If you live in a region infested with poisonous snakes, it is recommended that you get some snakebite kits. These are pocket-size and contain a suction device that eliminates the need to suck with your mouth.

Spine Fracture In the event of a fracture of the spine or dislocation of the back and neck, there will be deformation, possible cuts and bruises, and swelling. If the victim is conscious, you can ask whether he is suffering pain in the back or neck.

Look for cuts, bruises, and deformation. Feel along the back for tenderness to your touch. Check for paralysis of the neck by having the victim grasp your hand, raise his arms, and wiggle his fingers. To check for paralysis of the back, tickle the soles of the victim's feet to determine whether he has any feeling. Place your hand against his soles to see if he can push against your hand, and see if he can wiggle his toes.

If the victim is unconscious, look for cuts and bruises, and feel gently along the back for deformation. If possible, ask others what happened. With something pointed, gently jab the soles of the victim's feet or his ankles (to test for back injury) or hand (to test for neck injury). If the spinal cord is intact, the foot or hand should react.

A spine fracture or dislocation is difficult to diagnose in the unconscious victim. If the accident looks as though it could have produced a spinal injury, treat for one even though there are no other signs.

If the victim's neck may have been or certainly is fractured:
• Do not allow his head to be bent forward or backward, or from side to side. If the victim is having difficulty breathing, the airway has to be cleared but this must be done with extreme care lest a neck fracture be increased.
• If the victim is lying on his back, a small pad or towel may be placed in the space under his neck. But *do not* put a pillow under his head.
• Place rolled-up clothing or blankets around the victim's head, the sides of his neck, and his shoulders to prevent movement.
• Send for emergency services.

If the victim's back may have been or certainly is fractured:
1. Handle as little as possible.
2. Send for emergency services.
3. Until help arrives, leave the victim in the position in which he was found. Unless there is a delay in the arrival of an

ambulance, or his condition is critical, take care of all other emergencies – such as breathing difficulty, hemorrhage, and open wounds, applying dressings as necessary.

CAUTION

Do not twist the neck or back of a person who may have suffered a spine fracture.

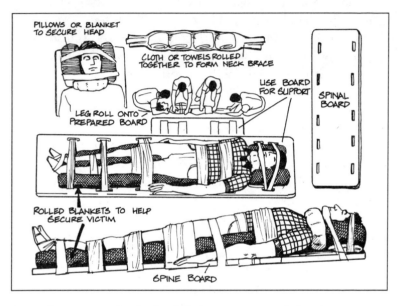

Spine fractures can be fatal or life-damaging. Immobilize the patient to prevent any movement. Never let his neck twist. And only attempt this if no emergency help is available.

Arrange rolled-up clothing or blankets on both sides of the body, head, and neck to immobilize the victim. If he must be turned to get his airway open (if he is, for example, face down in water or mud), it is essential that you get enough help so that his entire body is turned as a unit and no part twists or turns faster than another part.

Sprains A sprain results when ligaments or other tissues around joints are torn or stretched. The signs are pain during movement, swelling, and discolouration. The injured part should be elevated and cold compresses applied. Treat the sprain as you would a **fracture**. To be on the safe side, treat all injuries to the bones and joints as fractures.

Stings (See **Bites**)

Strains Strains are caused by overstretching a muscle or a tendon. Intense pain, moderate swelling, and difficulty in moving about without pain are the outward signs of such an injury. Apply mild, dry heat – and rest.

Stroke Stroke is caused by a blood clot or rupture of a blood vessel in the brain. The victim usually falls unconscious. His face usually will appear flushed and warm, but may sometimes appear ashen grey. His pulse will be slow and strong at first, then become rapid and weak later on. His respiration will be slow and will be accompanied by snoring sounds. The pupils will be of unequal size and there will be paralysis on one side of his face and/or body.

Make sure the victim's airway is open. Do not allow his tongue or saliva to block the air passage. Keep him warm, placing him in a semi-reclining position if his breathing is satisfactory. Keep him quiet and, if he is conscious, reassure him. Call for emergency medical assistance.

Unconsciousness There are hundreds of possible causes of unconsciousness, and you must check first to see that the victim is breathing.

CAUTION

Be careful in approaching an unconscious person to make sure that he is not in contact with electric current. If he is, turn off the electricity at the main switch or pull the plug, or if neither is possible, move the electrical wire away with a dry stick. (See pages 125-126.)

Try to awaken the victim. Shake his shoulder vigorously and ask him in a shouting voice if he is all right. If you get no response, check for signs of breathing.

Place him on his back, turning his head with the rest of his body so as not to bring about a neck injury. Loosen tight clothing around the neck, chest, and waist.

If there are no signs of neck or head injury, tilt the neck gently with one hand, causing the chin to protrude upward. Push down and back on the forehead with the other hand as you tip the head back. Now place an ear close to the victim's mouth and listen for sounds of breathing. Watch his chest and stomach for movement for at least 5 seconds.

If there is any question in your mind, or if breathing is so faint that you are unsure, assume the worst. Start **artificial respiration** immediately and have someone else call emergency services.

Wounds (See **Closed Wounds** and **Open Wounds**)

Preparing for the Unexpected

EFFECTIVE HANDLING of a medical emergency requires preparing for it before it occurs. Your home should have at least one first-aid kit. It should have a list of emergency telephone numbers pasted inside the lid and should contain, at minimum, the following items:

- Thermometer (oral and, if required, rectal)
- Rubbing alcohol
- Hydrogen peroxide
- Adhesive dressings (Band-Aid type) of all sizes
- One dozen individually wrapped sterile gauze pads (2" x 2"; or 5.1 cm x 5.1 cm)
- Six individually wrapped sterile gauze pads (4" x 4"; or 10 cm x 10 cm)
- Six non-stick sterile pads (2" x 4"; or 4.8 cm x 7.3 cm)
- One roll 2" (5 cm) gauze bandage
- One roll 5" (10 cm) gauze bandage
- Elastic (Ace-type) bandages (2" and 3"; or 5 cm and 7.5 cm)
- One triangular bandage (1 sq. yd; or 1 sq. m), muslin, folded diagonally
- Pair small scissors
- Pair pointed tweezers
- Aromatic spirits of ammonia
- Bottle of calamine lotion

- Box of baking soda
- Ice bag
- Epsom salts
- Syrup of ipecac
- Eye patches

You should also keep handy several old blankets and old clean pieces of sheeting stored in plastic bags to keep them clean and dust free.

Index

Concerning Children (*See also* Index of Symptoms)

Important Dos and Don'ts

Emergency Supply Requirements

Index of Symptoms

Acknowledgements

THE AUTHOR AND PUBLISHER acknowledge the assistance of material made available by the following:

Con Edison Department of Consumer Education

Committee on Accident Prevention, American Academy of Pediatrics

Emergency Planning Canada

National Institute for Occupational Safety and Health

Ontario Hydro Corporate Communications

Ontario Hydro Safety Services

Pickering Energy Information Centre

The Queen's Printer

Subcommittee on Accidental Poisoning, American Academy of Pediatrics

United States Printing Office